Swell-Wimp

Swell-Wimp

Sexual Exercise as a Means of Reducing

and Controlling Weight

Dr. Perry Bathous
Dr. Clarissa Flanders

toExcel
San Jose · New York · Lincoln · Shanghai

Swell-Wimp

This edition published by toExcel Press,
an imprint of iUniverse.com, Inc.

For information address:
iUniverse.com, Inc.
620 North 48th Street
Suite 201
Lincoln, NE 68504-3467
www.iUniverse.com

ISBN: 1-58348-735-2

Printed in the United States of America

First Preface

The weight loss and fitness program this book describes, Swell-Wimp, is the result of three occurrences. **(1)** While studying for my degree, a colleague and friend remarked that making love made her sweat—like a workout.[1] This caused me to wonder about how much work sexual partners perform—that is, how many calories are consumed. During the next year, I did some research and discovered that no serious work had been done on this subject.[2] I was unable to find even a calorie-per-type-of-exercise table that included sexual intercourse.[3] But with little time to spare during my internship, I put the project aside and eventually forgot about it.

(2) Several years later, while doing research for another project, I discovered that someone whom I admired immensely—Emily Dickinson—had brought her weight problem under control through will power and sexual exercise (see Appendix B). (3) While watching a video of the 1990 film, *Crazy People*, which exposes the duplicity of the advertising industry, an acquaintance[4] noticed that I had "put on a few pounds," and joked that I must not be "getting any." The remark was crude, but it reminded me of the comment my other friend had made and my earlier interest in the subject. I was then in a position to pursue the matter, so I began research in earnest.[5] Despite many difficulties and with the help of Dr. Flanders, the research has continued. This book is the result. I must admit that I am a Swell-Wimp apostle; I have personally benefited from the program.

I am grateful to the many people who made this book possible. In addition to my co-author and *socius criminis,* Dr. Clarissa Flanders, I would like to recognize four people who participated in our study—Harriet, Emily, Louisa and Fanny[6]—and the many contributions of George Tylutki, our editor.

Dr. Perry Bathous

Second Preface

When Dr. Bathous first discussed sexual exercise with me, it seemed a moronic idea. He invited me to take part in the study. He is very eloquent and persuasive, but I was skeptical (as you probably are) and I declined. A short time later, he again propositioned me. His preliminary results had been encouraging, but he was having difficulty obtaining resources. He pointed out the rewards that might be gained from the research. I became co-director of the study and was able to help him.

To not a small degree I am embarrassed to be associated with this book, not because of anything that is obscene or immoral, but because there are more important and urgent problems than weight loss. In the United States there are more than 30,000 metric tons of spent, radioactive, nuclear fuel stored at nuclear power plants and 2,000 more metric tons are created each year but no permanent nuclear waste repository exists nor is one scheduled to open before 2015. The number of cases of hypospadias, a birth defect, has doubled in the last 20 years. Of the world's three billion people about half live without clean toilets and two million children die each year from diarrhea-causing diseases. UNICEF estimates that providing world-wide sanitation would cost $68 billion spread over 10 years; that's only $680 million each year. Yet these issues (and many others) are generally ignored while the citizens of the United States alone spend $1.4 billion each year on treadmills![1]

Still, it cannot be denied that obesity is a significant problem which, at least, reduces quality of life and, at worst, leads to death. Swell-Wimp *does* work: it can result in weight loss and contribute to weight maintenance. It's easy, inexpensive and natural, and it's pleasurable. For these reasons I believe that Swell-Wimp is the only weight-loss/weight-maintenance program that a substantial number of people are likely to adopt and, more importantly, stay with. One can hope that as more and more Swell-Wimpers cease to be obese they will focus their time, energy and resources on other problems.

This is Perry's book; the idea was his and he did most of the research and writing. Despite his generous statement of gratitude, my contribution was limited. I would like to single out for recognition Mr. Norbert, Mr. Barville, Mr. Tylutki and especially Dr. Phil Tama, a dear friend and tireless researcher, who helped alleviate the many headaches the study occasioned.

Dr. Clarissa Flanders

Third Preface

This book is both a scientific report of our findings and a personal account. This may seem to be contradictory, but we want to present our findings as objectively as possible so that you and the scientific community can judge for yourselves. **And,** having benefited in several ways, we can testify to the rewards of sexual activity as part of an exercise and weight maintenance program.

You will, therefore, find a mixture of scientific discourse and plain speech. Where appropriate, we will explain any terms with which you may not be familiar. At the same time, we will not be prudish; we will not beat about the bush nor wallow in euphemisms (as Gore Vidal does when he writes of a man with a "rehnquist between his legs but no powells"); we will speak plainly and call a membrum virile a penis. As Giovanni Boccaccio says, "…there is nothing so unchaste but may be said chastely if modest words are used; …if there are a few words rather freer than suits the prudes [in this book]…I say that I should no more be reproved for having written them than other men and women are reproved for daily saying 'hole,' 'peg,' 'mortar,' 'pestle,' 'sausage,' 'Bologna sausage,' and the like things. My pen should be allowed no less power than is permitted the painter's brush".[1] We believe that *nihil obstat quominus imprimatur* our book. You will find nothing salacious or titillating herein; this is not a book to be read with one hand.

For those of you who are suspicious of anything shallow, artificial, low-quality, or insincere, we can assure you that our program is as comfortable as a cotton shirt, as reliable as a Volvo, and as natural as bean sprouts.

This book may change your life. It may make you think. Or it may only entertain you. But if you read it carefully, you can be sure that it will alter your view of sexual activity and exercise.

Dr. Perry Bathous
Dr. Clarissa Flanders

Acknowledgments

We owe much to the pioneers in this field, the men and women who have laid the groundwork for our study, such as Richard von Krafft-Ebing, Havelock Ellis, John Cleland, William H. Masters and Virginia E. Johnson,[1] Laurence Stern, Alfred C. Kinsey,[2] Wilt Chamberlain, Margaret Sanger, Cyrano de Bergerac, Katharine Davis, Marie Stopes, David Reuben, John Humphrey Noyes, Theodore van de Velde, June Reinisch, John Stith Pemberton, Shere Hite, Margaret Rudkin and, of course, Betty.

Of the following foundations, corporations and philanthropic organizations—Johnson & Johnson, Union Center for Women, National Organization for Women, British Museum, National Public Radio, MacArthur Foundation, Institute for Sex Research at Indiana University, Washington University Medical School, *Playboy,* Rockefeller Foundation, Carnegie Foundation, National Endowment for the Arts, Weight Watchers, Corporation for Public Broadcasting, Amway, National Science Foundation, Pennsylvania Higher Education Association, National Education Association, and the American Association of University Professors—none contributed funds or aid of any sort to our study.

We would very much like to make the information contained in this book available to everyone at no cost. However, we have received no corporate or foundation funding (yet). Much of the study was supported by individual (personal) contributions. Since we've had no more luck than Laurence Sterne at obtaining "fifty guineas," we very much need the proceeds from the sale of this book.

Quandoque bonus dormitat Homeros.[3] The several people who helped us with this book are not responsible in any way for its errors, inconsistencies or inaccuracies. They are our own.

Contents

Introduction

One might describe this book, not as *Insigne, recens, indictum ore alio,* but as *Non nova sed nove.*[1] It contains no discoveries or breakthroughs regarding dieting or sexual activity. Rather, we look at these in a new way.

Every action of the human body uses energy—walking, driving a car, waving bye-bye, blowing your nose, and so on. Some actions expend more energy than others—carrying a refrigerator upstairs versus making a bed. And sexual activity expends energy.

Most forms of exercise (the human body in action) in which people engage to lose or maintain weight are unpleasant—lifting weights, running, riding a stationary bicycle, and calisthenics, for example. But sexual activity is pleasant (to say the least).

Today, there are many Well-Wimps (**WE**ight **L**oss and We**I**ght **M**aintenance **P**rograms) being promoted, but most advocate unnatural forms of exercise or extreme diets. It is not natural for humans to run (except when fleeing from danger), to bat a ball over an artificial barrier (tennis), to pretend they are walking uphill in their living rooms (treadmills), or to jump up and down smacking their hands together over their heads (except when afflicted by some psychological disorder). Sexual activity is natural. In this book you will learn about a method of losing and/or maintaining weight through sexual activity.[2]

We call our program Swell-Wimp—**S**exual **WE**ight **L**oss and We**I**ght Maintenance Program. It can be used to lose weight or to maintain your weight and fitness. It can also enable you to occasionally indulge yourself (see Chapter 3). Today, book stores are overflowing with self-help books and cassette programs, such as Kalam Fadi's simplistic *Twelve Steps to Self-Confidence* (Riyadh: Rawis, 1988), the sweeping *The Eightfold Road to Enlightenment* by Siddhattha Gotama (Calcutta: Kalutas and Ganikas, 1982) and the ephemeral *The New Age Approach to Regularity* by A. Perient (NY: Yakov Andreyich Imprints, 1989). As you will see, *Swell-Wimp* does not belong to this category of self-help books. Swell-Wimp is not so much a

1

"program" with specific activities scheduled at certain times, but a more-or-less coherent set of guidelines.

Soon after my friend made the joke about my not "getting any," I was fortunate to meet someone uniquely qualified to help me with my research—Clarissa Flanders. Together we have perused the literature, conducted studies, interviewed subjects and run computer analyses. Ours is the most comprehensive study of its kind.[3] Swell-Wimp is the result.

A scene of the now-cancelled TV show *Reasonable Doubts*[4] opened with Dickie (Mark Harmon) and a lady friend in bed. Having arrived at the point of sexual climax, both are huffing and puffing. Afterward she says, "Want to do it again," and he answers that he couldn't handle the weight loss. Well, there you go; that's Swell-Wimp. The idea of using sexual activity to lose weight may sound silly, but it isn't. The idea has occurred to a number of people, but we have taken it seriously and studied it scientifically.

On National Public Radio's *All Things Considered*,[5] there was a report about the book *What Counts: The Complete Harper's Index*, edited by Charis Conn and Ilena Silverman. They pointed out that an extremely passionate kiss consumes 26 calories and a Hershey's Kiss contains 25 calories; so you could cancel the effects of eating Hershey's Kisses by kissing! However, instead of just tossing out some interesting numbers, we have investigated our subject deeply.

Finally, in an anti-smoking public service message on WCLH,[6] the speaker says that his wife said they could make love whenever he wanted to smoke. He goes on to say that (having quit smoking) he now feels much better and his wife and he have lost 160 pounds. We don't make such extravagant claims; 160 pounds is absurd. In this book we put forward a scientific and systematic method for increasing caloric expenditure during sexual activity in order to lose a moderate number of pounds in a reasonable time. If you want or need to "take 'em off," then "get it on."

Today, there is a tendency to rush to publish (because of academic pressures and the desire for fame and wealth) and to "publish" in the mass media instead of peer-reviewed journals. Failure to review one's findings, to replicate experiments and duplicate results can lead to disaster, as was seen in the case of our colleagues Pons and Fleishman. We believe in this system (peer review, not cold fusion, about which we have no firm opinion). But, sometimes scientists must bring their studies to a premature halt when it becomes obvious that a great harm is being done by not publishing the interim results; a tested medication, for example, demonstrates significant benefits such that it would be a crime of omission not to make the data available sooner rather than later. We feel compelled to publish before our studies are completed. Disciples of the Malignant Deity[7] of Nova Zembla[8] take note: it is true that publication may help us to obtain funding for continuing our studies, but that is not the sole or even primary reason for publishing at this point.

Academic and scientific journals can take a year or more to publish an article (especially if the editor is not convinced of the importance of the subject). It takes at least a year to get a traditional book published (most publishers won't even look at a manuscript unless it comes through an agent or is accompanied by a letter of recommendation from a best-selling author or Nobel Prize winner). There are a few popular magazines that would have published our study results but they do not have the authority necessary for our recommendations to be taken seriously and it would have been difficult if not impossible to explain Swell-Wimp in a brief article. So we chose electronic book publishing: it's fast, high-quality and inexpensive.

This book was composed quickly. We make no claim that it is comprehensive, although we have endeavored to include in it the results of the very latest research. Electronic publishing techniques have enabled us to revise, delete and insert material (primarily through the notes) virtually up to the day it was finalized. However, due to factors beyond our control, we were not able to do a complete re-editing of the book as a whole. You may find things a bit of a jumble in places; we apologize for any lack of coherence.

Chapter 1

Ad augusta per angusta[1]

Most of the participants in our study lost weight. Some gained strength and stamina. All became fitter—physically and sexually. Several ceased to be wimps (male or female). And they enjoyed the activities. Alex Comfort points out that "sexual exercise tones you better than jogging"—and wouldn't you rather?[2] If you adhere to the guidelines set forth in the following chapters, you will probably not become a Charles (or Charlene) Atlas, but no one will kick the bed covers in your face either. But, because each person's anatomy and physiology, attitudes, sense of humor, inclinations, degree of literacy, likes and dislikes are different, we cannot and do not make any specific claims for Swell-Wimp.

Dieting and Fitness Programs

You may be disappointed by the last sentence. We have all read the claims made on the covers of magazines at check-out counters[3]: "New electronic device flattens tummies in 2 minutes!"; "Lose 5 pounds a week eating only facial tissues!"; "The cabbages-and-strings diet melts pounds away!"[4] Swell-Wimp exercises alone won't make you slim and trim. After all, there are lots of fat[5], sexually-active people. You must, at least, keep your level of activity and eating at their current levels (if not higher and lower respectively). If you do so and engage in Swell-Wimp regularly, you will lose weight the proper way—slowly—and you will become fitter. Numerous studies have shown that only cutting calories (dieting) rarely works and that slow weight loss is less harmful and more likely to result in permanent weight reduction.[6] [7]

In fact, we don't make any claims for Swell-Wimp.[8] We have benefited from Swell-Wimp and hope that you will too, but we cannot guarantee it. Since you are reading this book, it is likely that you have read other "diet" books and may have taken part in weight-loss programs (for which extravagant claims were made). And you may have failed. You may even have a history of weight-loss failure. You may be overweight and weak-willed and you may have received a lot of negative feedback. How can we assure you that you will achieve fitness?

Or maybe you have never tried an exercise or weight-loss program before. You don't know what to expect and you are probably not prepared for the inevitable disappointments that will occur. For example, after an initial substantial weight reduction, subsequent pounds are more difficult to lose and it can be frustrating when again and again the scale does not greet you with good news. If this is your first attempt at exercise, you are a bad risk; that is, statistics show that most first-timers give up quickly. Statistics also show that repeat dieters and exercisers show substantial early success, but poor long-term results.[9]

Keys to Success

Stop! Don't put this book down yet. *Nil desperandum*: things are not hopeless. Not at all. Many people do achieve success when engaging in an exercise or dieting program. Why do some succeed and so many fail? There are two[10] factors: (1) the weight-loss/weight-maintenance program and (2) the exerciser/dieter.

The Program

There is not much to say about the importance of the program to success; it is both crucial and irrelevant. That is, any program that aims toward fitness through long-term exercise and diet control without disrupting normal daily activities is a good program. Swell-Wimp is a good program.

A successful program must change the way you live, slowly and permanently. For example, you must stop eating too much, stop eating the wrong kinds of food and/or frequently engage in some type of pleasurable exercise that will keep you trim and fit. Although the number of calories you eat is important, their source is more significant. Calories obtained from fat sources (ice cream, for example) are more likely to cause you to put on weight than those derived from carbohydrates. There are many activities that dieters do not stick with over the long term—eating grapefruit three times a day, wearing plastic wrap, and running miles and miles before breakfast.[11] These just do not become a part of normal daily life.[12] It is not normal or natural to run for fun or pretend that you are rowing a boat in your bedroom. Thus, the wrong kind of program is almost certain to fail (except for fanatics) and the right kind of program is almost certain to succeed (except for the truly hopeless). Our program belongs in the latter category.

In the last two decades the average American's working hours have increased by one month per year.[13] The United States is now #1 of the industrialized nations for the number of hours the average worker works. This means that you have less time for leisure activities and exercise, and you probably have less money (in real terms). Less time and less money for exercise—what to do? Swell-Wimp is inexpensive compared to health-club fees and the cost of golf clubs.[14] Swell-Wimp is convenient. You don't have to drive to the golf course or health-club (although you may have to travel to meet your partner). You can do it at night and in bad weather. You can do it without a lot of planning.

More and more people are exercising alone at home using videos. I have before me a brochure that came in the mail, *The Complete Guide to Exercise Videos*. It describes videos for doing dance aerobics to various kinds of music: country, rock, hula, funk, hip hop, soul, macarena and gospel.[15] There are videos for high impact, low impact, stretch and step aerobics and for using freeweights, shaper balls, jump ropes, slide pads, swimming pools, steps and even chairs. There are videos for firming, toning, reducing, sculpting and enhancing abs, buns, thighs, the upper body, the middle body, the lower body, and the total body and for building bones. There are exercise videos involving Kung-Fu, Tai Chi, Chi Kungyoga, kickboxing, ballet and calisthenics. There are videos for pregnant women, arthritics, kids and senior citizens (and everyone in between).[16]

The cover of the brochure proclaims "Convenient. Private. Fun." The first two claims may be true, but is the third? Certainly all three apply to Swell-Wimp. And we might add "Inexpensive. Natural." Except for those aimed specifically at children, all of the videos could be replaced with Swell-Wimp.[17] Unlike most videos and self-help books, we will show you how to engage in a normal, natural and pleasurable activity in a programmatic manner so as to develop and maintain fitness. You can continue to do it as long as you live. And it is equally easy, pleasurable and effective for both men and women.[18]

The Program Participant

The second and most important, factor in determining whether you successfully lose weight is you. If your attitude is good, you will probably succeed; if not, you won't.[19] You must understand that losing weight requires expending energy which is work (although with Swell-Wimp it is pleasurable work to be sure). Pounds do not "melt" away and you cannot achieve muscle tone "without effort." "Keeping the weight off" is harder than losing it, because you must alter your lifestyle to some extent; you must learn to eat less and differently and to exercise more. *Consilio Manuque*.[20] Finally, you must be prepared for some relapses.

But, as the Surrealists say, "Large birds make little Venetian blinds." The mind is a powerful thing. David Reuben calls the brain the most important sexual organ.[21] The mind can hold us back. William Blake in his famous poem about eighteenth-century London blames the horrible conditions on "mind-forg'd manacles" (mental handcuffs): people's attitudes prevented them (harlots, children, soldiers) from improving their situations. And in "Chains of Love," the singers claim that the chains "got a hold on me" but aren't the "kind that you can see": the attitude/emotion we call love can enslave us to others. The mind can also enable us to do great things: the ant was able to move the rubber-tree plant because he had "high hopes." So you must **want** to lose weight. You must feel that you **can** lose weight. And you must be determined that you **will** lose weight.[22]

Attitude is crucial! Whether this is the first time or the tenth time that you have tried to lose weight, you MUST BELIEVE you can achieve your goal. When you stop thinking of yourself as just **A** person and begin seeing yourself as an **I**ndividual—a valuable and capable **I**—then f**A**t becomes f**I**t.

Most readers and critics think of the great American poet, Emily Dickinson, as a virginal recluse whose major themes were renunciation, death, and nature. This is true, but she was also a modern and passionate person and her poetry is very personal and erotic. Few people realize that Emily's shyness and insecurity were, in part, the result of her struggle with obesity.[23] In Poem 351 she says:

> I felt my life with both my hands
> I turned my Being round and round
> And paused at every pound
> I judged my features—jarred my hair—
> I pushed my dimples by, and waited—

> I told my self, "Take Courage, Friend—
> That—was a former time—"

Through will power and sexual activity she eventually overcame her weight problem. What she wrote about sexual relations, personal appearance and attitude is still relevant and useful and we will be quoting her occasionally. You may want to read Appendix B now because her life and work give great encouragement to Swell-Wimpers.[24]

Feedback Loops

There are no miracle cures for obesity nor easy roads to fitness. You have to break old patterns of improper eating and avoiding exercise and replace them with new, healthier patterns.[25] You must be determined, have patience and take charge of your body and your life. Slowly and steadily (despite setbacks) you will see results—and so will others. Their attitudes will change as they see their "fat friend" become self-confident and sexy. And even though your hair may turn gray, they will see that you remain trim, energetic and desirable.[26] Swell-Wimp works because it is fun, because it helps you to change your attitudes, and because it is by definition a long-term program.

There are natural feedback loops[27] in Swell-Wimp. As you lose weight, you feel better about your appearance. You want your partner(s) to see your new body. You feel sexier and project sexiness, and, thus, become more desirable to your partner(s). So, you engage in sexual exercise more frequently which results in losing more weight and feeling even better about yourself and so on. This doesn't really happen with other kinds of exercise; becoming more desirable to your partner doesn't usually lead to more time with the Thigh Master.

There is another feedback loop. Heat production is proportional to body mass (the amount of muscle available to generate heat) which increases with the cube of linear dimensions, such as your height. However, heat loss is proportional to body surface (the amount of skin available to release the heat) which increases only with the square of your linear dimensions. The more mass you have, the more heat you generate. The more skin surface you have, the more heat you lose. Thus, fat people feel hotter and can withstand the cold more. So, as you lose weight you keep almost the same skin surface area and reduce the number and size of the adipose deposits; therefore, you feel cooler. Because you feel cooler (and are, in fact, cooler), you can exercise more. This results in more weight loss and the loop is reinforced.

Further, as you continue Swell-Wimp, lose weight and become fitter, you are capable of doing more "work" for longer periods and more frequently. And, as your body gets smaller, you can do things you couldn't before: you can bend down and tie your shoes or assume a difficult sexual position. Being able to do more work, you DO more work. Doing more work means burning more calories and losing more weight and so on.[28] This is also true of other forms of exercise but being able to ride a stationary bicycle for longer periods seems a punishment, not a positive reinforcement.

Interestingly, obesity can cause impotence in men.[29] Thus, as you do Swell-Wimp, your impotence probably will become less severe and/or less frequent.[30] This will make you a better sexual partner and you will expend more energy, thus losing more weight in another feedback loop.

Finally, because Swell-Wimp is performed with a partner there is another kind of feedback that doesn't occur if you exercise alone. You keep an eye on each other, making sure the other is exercising. When you see your partner working, sweating, feeling tired and sore, you know you are not alone. As you see your partner losing weight and becoming sexier, you are encouraged to go on. You benefit as your partner becomes more sexually skilled, and your partner benefits as you become sexier and more skilled. To paraphrase Langston Hughes, boink and be boinked in return. You compliment and encourage each other. This doesn't happen as you run a treadmill alone and you certainly don't gain pleasure each time you exercise.

Physical Examination

Before you begin Swell-Wimp, you and your partner(s) should have a complete physical examination by a qualified health-care professional for four reasons. First, during orgasm, a person's heart rate can zoom to 160 beats per minute and his or her blood pressure can double. Sex puts a strain on the body! Swell-Wimp is not a strenuous program nor is it dangerous, but as lawyers say, *"praemonitus praemunitus"* (forewarned, forearmed). If you have a condition of any sort that prevents you from engaging in exercise, you should not begin Swell-Wimp. You need to know that your sexual, cardiovascular, and other systems are, at least, normal. And you need to have an accurate measurement of your weight before beginning Swell-Wimp (bathroom scales are notoriously inaccurate).

Second, a physical examination may reveal conditions which could mask the results of Swell-Wimp. For example, if you were pregnant or had a tumor (benign, it is to be hoped), it might appear that you were actually GAINING weight. This could lead to disappointment, even depression. Or, conversely, some medical conditions might cause you to lose weight and the fact that you were engaging in exercise would mask that condition; you would probably be pleased that you were losing so much weight so quickly (not knowing that you were ill). Inattention to any medical condition can lead to serious consequences, so get an exam before you begin.

Third, you need to know if you have any communicable, especially sexually-transmitted, diseases or conditions such as syphilis, gonorrhea, lice, Gongorism, genital herpes, chlamydia trachometis, aegra omans, chiliasm, AIDS, atrabilious schadenfreude, molluscum contagiosum, aura popularis, granuloma inguinale, nudum pactum, lymphogranuloma venereum, mesokurtic Neozapatismo, Fungoso, viral hepatitis, Kortgatsyndroem, Peyronis disease, or contagious tuberculosis.[31] You MUST NOT engage in sexual activity with another person if there is ANY possibility that you will transmit a disease to (or contract from) him or her. It is definitely immoral, and in some cases illegal, to do so. Ignorance is no defense. You should know. Further, finding out that you have such a disease will enable you to get treatment. Don't delude yourself by thinking that you couldn't possible have VD. If you are so sure, then you will not mind confirming it with an examination.[32]

Almost everyone now understands that AIDS is not a disease of only drug users and homosexuals. Peter Radetsky reports that at least 70% of the people in the world infected with HIV caught it from their heterosexual partners.[33] Certain types of sexual activity are more risky than others because they involve direct contact with body fluids: for example, anal intercourse, intercourse during menstruation, and swallowing semen. Many people cannot say with 100% certainty that they do not carry the HIV virus,[34] because a substantial amount of time can pass between the time of exposure to the virus and its detection. Because AIDS IS INCURABLE and because you are unlikely to require a blood test and complete social and medical history of your sexual partner(s), you MUST BE CAREFUL. If either partner is a carrier of the AIDS virus, then there is virtually no safe sexual activity for them except mutual masturbation while wearing gloves.

You can reduce your chances of contracting AIDS by avoiding partner(s) who are members of high-risk groups: those who have had direct contact with blood and other body fluids (intravenous drug users, prostitutes, surgeons, proctologists, elementary-school teachers, phlebotomists, and ex-drug users) and those who have had many partners. Sex with long-term partners (life-long is best) is safer than with short-term partners. If you have tested positive for the HIV virus, you should have sex only with others who have also tested positive and inform all of your partners that you have tested positive. You can reduce the risk of contracting AIDS by using condoms, but complete abstinence from sexual activity is the surest method.

Using condoms only partially reduces your risk of being infected by a human papilloma virus, the most common, sexually-transmitted infection in the US and Europe (because it can live in the outer skin as well as within the vagina, cervix, urethra and anus). Several of these viruses can cause cancer, yet the infection produces no immediate, obvious symptoms.

There is just so much stuff going around nowadays in addition to AIDS that you can be sure that you are not infected with papilloma, gonorrhea or syphilis, for example, only by being examined.[35] Poverty is no excuse; there are public hospitals, free clinics, and other institutions/organizations that you can go to. Further, weeks or months may pass between the time you are infected and the time symptoms begin to appear; so you should be examined periodically, especially if you have more than one sexual partner or your partner has more than one partner. For more about AIDS see Chapters 9 and 13.

Fourth, you need to have a physical examination in order to protect us, the authors (*caveat venditor*).[36] If you came to us to get into our Swell-Wimp program, we would examine you first. But we can't do that because we are talking to you through this book, not face-to-face. It would be unfair of you to begin Swell-Wimp without an examination and then have a heart attack. People would ask "How did it happen?" and when told that you were taking part in the Swell-Wimp program, they would suspect that Swell-Wimp caused the heart attack. The program would get a bad name. Some of your friends and relatives might even want to sue us, thinking that we were responsible for your injury, when, of course, it would have been your own lack of concern for yourself and others that hurt you.

So, let us say again: You MUST have a complete physical examination BEFORE beginning Swell-Wimp. You MUST NOT begin Swell-Wimp if there is any indication that you have a communicable disease. You MUST NOT begin Swell-Wimp if the examination indicates that you have a condition that might result in harm to yourself (or others) if you engage in the activities described in the following pages. Be sure to read the entire book before beginning Swell-Wimp. The exercises and instructions in this book are not substitutes for medical counseling and common sense. **NEITHER THE AUTHORS NOR THE PUBLISHERS WILL BE LIABLE FOR ANY LOSS OR INJURY TO ANY PARTY IN CONNECTION**

WITH THE RECOMMENDATIONS, SUGGESTIONS, INSTRUCTIONS OR ADVICE HEREIN CONTAINED.

As you read this book, you may occasionally feel that we are belaboring the obvious. However, it was recently reported in the newspapers that a woman said she could not understand how she got AIDS since she always took her birth control pills. It's clear that the woman who thought birth control pills would protect her from AIDS, didn't know how a person contracts AIDS or the limitations of oral contraceptives. If, as you are reading, it seems that we are explaining things that everybody already knows, remember this woman. And feel some sympathy for her. A little knowledge might have helped her. None of us knows everything and too many of us know too little.[37] We do not intend to insult your intelligence; we are simply trying to give everybody as much knowledge as possible.

As mentioned before, our study was not completed: this is really an interim report. As such it is not really a how-to book and is not meant for the lay person. However, the results of our investigations are so clear that we felt compelled to present them to the public at this time. It is our hope[38] to begin a new study in the near future from which we expect to be able to develop new exercise activities and methods, a better understanding of why men lose more weight (short-term) than women, and obtain long-term data. At the conclusion of that study, we will publish our findings in a series of articles in the appropriate journals and publish a more comprehensive and coherent book for the public.

In the meantime, read on to learn about Swell-Wimp, the Sexual Weight Loss and Weight Maintenance Program. It's easy, it's natural and it's fun.

Chapter 2

Work and Play: Sex Is Work

The human body converts the foods we eat into energy. If we take in more food-energy than we need, we gain weight because the excess is stored as fat. Metabolism is the name given to this complicated process of converting food into energy and storing the excess temporarily in some organs and long-term in adipose deposits. In addition to obtaining energy from food (derived from carbohydrates, starches, fats, sugars), the body extracts other necessary nutrients: proteins, vitamins, fats (yes, the body needs some fat), and minerals. Since the body can more easily store excess calories derived from fat (carbohydrate calories, for example, are not easily stored), you must be concerned with the kinds of food you eat (fruits, whole grains and carbohydrates are good; fats are bad) as well as the amounts.

Each individual's metabolism is different; some people "burn up calories" more quickly (easily) than others. But the variations among individuals are not large. There are those whose metabolism varies substantially from the norm, but they are not as common as many people think. That is, most fat people do not have a "gland problem"; they just take in more energy than they use and the excess is stored as fat.[1]

This is another reason for having a physical examination before beginning Swell-Wimp. You might learn that you are one of the rare people with a "gland problem." If so, you need medical care, because Swell-Wimp (nor any program of dieting/exercising) probably will not help you lose weight or firm up; in fact, it may do harm. Therefore, you must get a physical examination from a qualified health professional before beginning Swell-Wimp.

There are only three ways to lose weight. (1) When you **diet** you take in fewer calories by eating either (a) less food or (b) lower-calorie foods. (2) When you **exercise** (work) you "burn up" more calories by doing (a) more activities or (b) more strenuous activities. (3) In the third category are all of the unpleasant pharmaceuticals and procedures that circumvent the normal process of digestion and fat storage: lipo-suction, diuretics, laxatives, diet pills, vomiting, stomach stapling, etc. Swell-Wimp belongs in the second category and in later chapters we will be discussing how to engage in more sexual activities and more strenuous sexual activities. You should keep in mind that exercising won't help you lose weight (or maintain your weight) unless you also control your diet.

Dieting

Dieting decreases the amount of food-energy that you take in. There are two ways to do this: (1) eat less food (one pork chop instead of three) or (2) eat foods that con-tain less energy (lettuce instead of cream puffs). Of course, dieting is really more complicated than this. The body requires a daily minimum amount of vitamins, min-erals, protein, fat, etc.—a balanced diet. That is why you should avoid "fad diets" based on eating primarily one food (like grapefruit): improper diet can lead to nutri-tional deficiencies. You should be very skeptical of diets and weight-loss programs that appear in popular books and magazines. Sensible diets and dieting guidelines can be obtained from your physician, hospitals, dietitians, organizations like the American Heart Association and numerous national, state and even local govern-mental agencies. Ultimately though, reduced caloric intake by itself rarely results in long-term weight reduction.

When you diet, your body tries to conserve energy by slowing down your metab-olism because it must use some of your fat stores and thus it thinks that you are starv-ing. Ironically, you burn fewer calories because your metabolism is slower and thus, it is harder to lose weight. When you exercise, your metabolic rate increases in order to meet your exercising energy needs, and it is easier to burn fat and lose weight.[2] Therefore, it is more difficult to lose weight when you only diet (without exercise), than when you diet and exercise. More than one-half of the calories taken in are burned by basal metabolism—the energy rate needed simply to live (when we are at rest). Studies have shown that exercise increases basal metabolism, so when you reg-ularly exercise, you burn more calories even when you are not actively exercising. Further, even if exercising doesn't result in a loss of pounds, you may become trim-mer, because fat will be replaced by muscle which occupies less space.

Exercise

Exercising increases the number of calories you "burn up." There are two ways to do this: (1) increase the number of physical activities you engage in (for example, go for a walk after work) or (2) increase the strenuousness of the physical activities you engage in (for example, go for a run instead of a walk). Exercising is one of the best things you can do for yourself. Studies show that it offers protection against disease and death even in people whose risk factors—high blood pressure, for example—put them in danger. The chief benefits occur when you change from a sedentary lifestyle to one of moderate exercise,[3] not from moderate to extreme exercise. Swell-Wimp is moderate exercise.

While exercising, you use the energy the body has obtained from food.[4] If you expend more energy than the body has recently taken in, you will begin to deplete the body's energy stores (fat). It is easier to exercise than diet because you do not have to be knowledgeable about nutrients and such, but exercising is not risk free. You can injure yourself (pull a muscle, tear a ligament) or bring on a serious medical emergency (heart attack, heat stroke). Further, you will not achieve long-term fitness if you only exercise and give no thought to diet (for example, eating Twinkies while "pumping iron"). A proper weight-loss and weight-maintenance program includes diet and exercise management.

As was pointed out earlier, all physical activity uses energy. **Work** is the name we give to energy-using activities. Sweeping the floor, butchering a hog, and digging a ditch are all, obviously, work. But so are playing tennis, playing hide-and-seek, playing cards, playing the stock market, playing dead and foreplay. Those things we call "play" are actually work. That which distinguishes work from play is the amount of pleasure we obtain from the activity. Some people fish for a living and some do it for "fun." Some hate mowing the lawn and others enjoy it. Some kinds of play require large amounts of energy (a brisk game of tennis or basketball, mountain climbing, jumping rope) and some don't (chess, golf, kite flying, reading). Likewise, some kinds of work are energy intensive (professional football and teaching) and some are not (lawyering and legislating). There is no difference between work and play in terms of energy use; some people expend more energy playing than working.

Of course, simply living requires energy; our hearts pump, our digestive system digests, and so on (basal metabolism). We apply the term work to any activity (work or play) that requires energy use beyond the level necessary simply to maintain life.[5] Thus, showering is work. And going out for the mail is work. Changing channels with the remote control is also work. And sexual activity is work. This fact is at the heart of the Swell-Wimp program. Sexual activity is work; work uses energy; if energy use exceeds energy intake, weight loss occurs. ut;s sunoekl ut;s batyrak; abd ut;s fyb!xxxx xxxxxxx xxxx xxxxxxxx xxx xxxx xxxxIt's easy; it's natural; and it's fun!

Why has no one attempted to determine how many calories are used during various sexual activities and use that information to devise a program for weight loss and maintenance? There are several reasons. (1) Traditionally, sex was viewed as something dirty and nasty and thus not a proper subject of research. Kinsey's landmark study didn't appear until 1948 and even as late as that he encountered opposition from politicians, academics and religious.[6] (2) The idealized, romanticized view of sex also inhibited study. Thus, sex was seen as the high point of a mysterious process called love. The real essence of sex (the transformation of two into one, or something like that) was thought to have little to do with the physical. It was beyond study, like science trying to study beauty or honesty. (3) Compared to highly-physical activities (swimming, digging ditches, ball playing, branding cattle), sex is not an energy-intensive activity.[7] After all, from the male point of view it only took a few minutes and a real man could do it without even becoming winded.[8]

Few people saw sex as a very physical activity that feels really good. Apparently, it never crossed anyone's mind that sex could be part of a fitness program.[9] (1) Anyone interested in fitness and exercise would, therefore, look to obviously physical activities—calisthenics, running, weight lifting—that expend a lot of energy. (2) Most of us have a propensity to give more credence to things which have been formalized. We "know" we'll lose more weight if we must maintain a regular schedule, purchase special clothing and equipment, keep records and even go to meetings. (3) We believe that ordinary and routine things are not as effective as the unusual and special. If we have to go to a gym or pool or park to exercise, it must be better than simply using the stairs instead of the elevator, walking instead of driving, and so on. (4) Further, we "know" that anything that is good for us must be somewhat painful, distasteful, or unpleasant (and sex isn't any of these).[10]

So, we are the first to scientifically study the calorie-expending aspects of sexual activity and the first to provide the information necessary to lose weight or maintain weight through sexual activity. *Consumer Reports* in a report on dieting books says, "The boring truth is that a sensible diet, in combination with exercise, has always been the best way for most people to lose weight."[11] Well, the "truth" may be boring, but the exercise doesn't have to be if you use Swell-Wimp.

Definition

It is time that we define a term that we have been using for quite some time—sexual activity. When we use that term, we generally mean vaginal intercourse between a male and female. In addition to the actual act of intercourse,[12] we include activities generally known as foreplay and postplay,[13] such as kissing, stroking, rubbing, fellatio, and cunnilingus.

Throughout the rest of this book we will use the terms **SexAct** for sexual activity and **SexEx** (or *coitus exercisus*[14]) for sexual exercise. In addition to these activities, we will be discussing other items that can contribute to weight loss and fitness: attire, diet, equipment, special exercises, and more.

Caveats[15]

The human sexual life is rich and varied. Although we (the authors) may be personally disgusted by some sexual practices, it is not our place (as scientists) to make moral judgments. As the Romans said: *sua cuique voluptas* (different strokes for different folks). Attitudes about sexual matters have changed considerably in the last 25 years.[16] Still, we must write plainly about real things.[17] We do not advocate sexual promiscuity; we do advocate frequent and vigorous sexual activity to promote weight loss and weight maintenance.

Although we do discuss increasing the frequency of your sexual encounters, our primary emphasis is on expending more calories during each sexual activity. Even if you do increase the frequency, this does not automatically mean that you will have more partners. Swell-Wimp is a method of making more useful something you already do and enjoy. If you are celibate (for whatever reason), we do not urge you to become sexually active. If you are overweight and sexually active, we do not advocate that you seek additional partners. Sexual relationships are complex. For most people, sex is more than just physical and for some it is even spiritual. Sex is not a neutral activity; it involves ego, emotions, and your moral self. The pleasures of sex are accompanied by responsibilities;[18] some sexual activities can result in pregnancy and others can lead to physical damage and transmission of disease. Sex can even kill.

Traditionally, SexAct could have three purposes. The **first** was procreation. Even non-coital SexAct can result in conception; the male doesn't have to ejaculate into the female for sperm to be transferred. The bulbo-urethral glands[19] supply a few drops of secretion which appear shortly after erection and they contain many thousands of sperm. Thus, even prior to ejaculation the fluid that "leaks" from the penis contains sperm, and placing the penis in the vagina even without ejaculation can result in conception, pregnancy and years of child-care. It doesn't really matter how the sperm get there, so be careful! If you believe that procreation is the only reason for sexual relations, then Swell-Wimp is not for you.[20]

The **second** purpose was positive emotional/psychological interaction. People who like each other (traditionally, we have expected strong liking, even loving) do something they enjoy—together. This is just like playing cards or watching a movie, except that (1) the participants bear a greater responsibility to each other because conception may occur and (2) it is more pleasurable, which was the **third** purpose. Orgasm is very pleasurable. SexAct in which the second and third purposes occur together is even more pleasurable. SexAct in which the second is negative rather than positive is rape (or assault or batter or whatever it is called in your state). It is deplorable and requires counseling (at least) or incarceration. So, we are **not** saying "do it" whenever and wherever you can with whomever you want.

Now there is a **fourth** purpose for sexual relations: sex for exercise. Increasing the frequency and vigor with which you engage in safe sexual activity can lead to weight loss. If you are not overweight, but are approaching middle-age, Swell-Wimp can help you to avoid putting on pounds. And this fourth purpose relates to the other three. If you want it to, your SexEx can result in conception. Probably you will do it with someone you like. And it should be pleasurable.

So we will be objectively discussing a number of SexActs that some people may not be comfortable with.[21] Like Chaucer[22] and Boccaccio,[23] we are advising you here about the contents of the rest of the book. You will have to decide for yourself what you want—to lose excess pounds and maintain your weight (and read on) or adhere to old-fashioned sexual attitudes.[24] We should also point out here that unlike many other physical exercises, more intercourse is not necessarily better.[25] Any gains made by engaging in intercourse very frequently (for example, every sixty minutes) will be offset by decreased libido, disorientation and increased medical costs. We do not endorse or recommend "machine-gun" or "marathon" sex. Rather, regular, controlled, enhanced, informed SexEx is the key to long-term success. We will be discussing more frequent sexual activities and more strenuous sexual activities in the next chapter.

Also, you should **NOT** take anabolic steroids to improve your sexual performance. We will show later that strength is only one (and not the most important) aspect of SexEx. Further, sheer muscle mass will not improve performance and may, in fact, hinder it (remember the drowning, muscle-bound, body builder). Steroids do not improve stamina, sensitivity, agility, or flexibility; they may actually reduce these. Finally, they can lead to sterility, liver and kidney damage and priapism in males (see below).

When you lift weights, you work up to heavier and heavier lifts. When you run, you work up to longer distances or shorter times. Although Kinsey reports that high rates of sexual activity do not seem to contribute to physical impairment or other difficulties,[26] you should not think of Swell-Wimp in terms of performance—more, longer, deeper, faster. The aim should be to structure your SexActs for maximum pleasure and energy expenditure in order to increase fitness and achieve weight loss. There are no records to surpass nor prizes to win. So, you should not only NOT take steroids, but also not shave your head and/or body hair (including pubic hair) as swimmers do in order to enhance your performance.[27] It may, in fact, be detrimental, since you are likely to feel self-conscious and cold and your partner may not like it (especially, the stubble that will appear in a day or so).

The following chapters set forth a program of sexual activity between partners designed to help one or both lose or maintain weight. We do not directly address the needs of those who prefer objects or animals as sexual partners or of those who prefer multiple, simultaneous partners. However, they may find some of the information useful. Since the exercises described are related to opposite-partnered sexual intercourse, homosexuals (male or female) will have to extrapolate where applicable.[28] We do, however, discuss Swell-Wimp in relation to older people in Chapter 14.

We did not investigate (as far as we know) nor will we be discussing incest, necrophilia[29] or zoophilia,[30] brutal and demeaning sexual activities, such as bondage,[31] whipping, French Kissing, catachresis, Schneewittchen and other Sado-Masochistic practices, nor various paraphilias that generally do not lead to intercourse, such as fetishism, transvestism, epithalamia, pedophilia, apotemnophilia, coprophilia,[32] urophilia, frotteurism and so on.[33] These activities differ from other sexual practices primarily in the fact that they involve physical and/or psychological pain or transgression of societal sexual norms. Personally, we don't much care what you do as long as you do not hurt anyone:[34] you cause hurt if you have sex without the consent of the other as in rape and child molestation; you cause hurt if you have sex with someone who is not prepared as with a child, the physically and mentally incapable (whether due to congenital defect, injury or illness); you do harm if you have sex with someone who is intellectually, emotionally or psychologically unprepared (as with those whose beliefs prohibit sex); you cause harm when you injure another during sex, whether physical (hitting or passing on a disease, for example) or psychological (denigrating the other); and you cause hurt when you do harm after sex, by disparaging him or her afterwards, making the sexual activity known to others in spite of your partner's wishes, and so on. We believe that sex should be synonymous with pleasure; hurting has no place in Swell-Wimp.

Both Vatsyayana and the Marquis de Sade wrote about the role of pain in sexual pleasure. De Sade wrote for the individual who defies moral codes; he finds pain an ESSENTIAL ingredient of sexual pleasure. Vatsyayana finds it one of many possible contributors to sexual pleasure.[35] Some contemporary experts hold that the pain involved in such activities can be and is pleasurable to both the giver and receiver. Really? If you punch your employer, you may feel pleasure, but does he or she? Of course not. Your hand hurts, but the pleasure you receive is not derived from the pain in your hand. How can having your nipples pinched or your testicles squeezed be pleasurable?[36] If you enjoy such things, you will not find much in this book of interest. Nothing in this book should be construed as disparaging of persons who are sexually celibate (asexual) or prefer to confine their sexual activities to themselves (autoerotics).

Masturbation and Autoeroticism

Because of a lack of funds and the publication deadline, we were unable to investigate Swell-Wimp in relation to autoerotic sexual activity. Masturbation is a normal human activity; today we know that masturbation will not cause acne, venereal disease or the growth of hair on your hands. It's easy to look back and wonder how such claims could be made without any scientific basis, but we are not free of such ideas even today. We must always be critical and skeptical (in the positive sense) and be ever watchful for shoddy scholarship and absurd or inflated claims.[37]

Most people masturbate at some time[38] and many continue to do it frequently during their entire lives with no harmful effects.[39] In some situations—prison, war, mental hospital, extreme ugliness—it is often the only (legal) method of achieving sexual satisfaction.[40]

Kinsey reports that masturbation is the sexual outlet by which females most frequently achieve orgasm (95%), although intercourse is the one in which the largest number engage after marriage.[41] Shere Hite points out that masturbation increases a woman's ability "to orgasm"[42] in general and "to orgasm" during intercourse (189).

Emily Dickinson often engaged in masturbation when unable to arrange a meeting with her sexual partners. She writes about this in Poem 773:

> Deprived of other Banquet,
> I entertained Myself—
> At first—a scant nutrition—
> An insufficient Loaf—
> But grown by slender addings
> To so esteemed a size
> 'Tis sumptuous enough for me—
> And almost to suffice

For women who infrequently or never achieve orgasm during coitus, masturbation may be the best way to learn how—what needs to be stimulated, when and how much. And masturbation is useful for relieving sexual tension when your partner is unavailable for a period of time. It is one of the most frequent forms of sexual outlet among the elderly and handicapped.

If you prefer auto-sexual behavior, you can still practice Swell-Wimp. Keep in mind that you want to maintain or decrease your daily caloric intake. This can be a problem for females. For example, if you routinely eat your dildo, you should choose it carefully. A cucumber dildo is low in calories and high in vitamins and makes an excellent choice. A banana dildo, however, is high in calories and tooth-rotting sugars and a wiener dildo is high in fats, sodium and nitrates.[43]

We hope to study masturbation and investigate methods of making it more energy intensive. We can make some suggestions now: wear weights on your wrists, but regularly switch hands to avoid unilateral overdevelopment of the hand, shoulder and arm[44]; walk around while you do it (around the house or on a treadmill); wear lots of clothes to sweat or do it naked in a cold room to shiver (see Chapter 10 regarding heat and cold); repeatedly bring yourself to the brink of climax and then stop (see Chapter 5).

Sexual and Work Energy

Throughout the rest of this book, we will be using two terms: sexual energy and work energy. We are all familiar with work energy; this refers to the use of our voluntary muscles to play tennis, dig a hole or engage in coitus. Sexual energy is similar to nervous energy. When we are nervous, our hearts beat more quickly (involuntary muscle) and our muscles often tense (involuntary use of voluntary muscles). Sexual energy is expended when we are aroused and/or are engaged in SexEx. Our heart and respiration rates increase, certain muscles and muscle groups tense and/or contract and expand, and hormonal activity increases. Masters, Johnson and Kolodny report that there are two basic physiologic reactions during human sexual response: (1) vasocongestion, which is an increased amount of blood concentrated in body tissues in the genitals and female breasts; (2) myotonia or increased neuro-muscular tension, which is a buildup of energy in the nerves and muscles.[45] Sexual energy (a term we prefer to myotonia) accounts for only a small caloric expenditure, but it mounts up with regular and intense SexAct. You should not underestimate its role in Swell-Wimp.[46]

Chapter 3

FreqSex: Increasing Sexual Activity

The ancients used to say, *non est vivere sed nalere vita est*,[1] and being well means being healthy— fit and trim. As we pointed out earlier, there are two ways to lose weight: take in fewer calories (we discuss diet in a later chapter) or increase the number of calories expended (burned up). You can do this (1) by increasing the number of energy-expending activities you take part in: take up golf or gardening or golf or garden more frequently. Engaging in SexAct more often we call FreqSex (more **Freq**uent **Sex**ual activity). (2) Alternatively, you can engage in more strenuous activities: switch from golf to weight lifting or from gardening to chopping wood. Engaging in sexual activities that expend more energy we call StrenSex (for more **Stren**uous **Sex**ual activity). In this chapter we focus on FreqSex— specifically, engaging in SexAct more frequently. In later chapters, we discuss making SexAct more strenuous. Of course, if you engage in both StrenSex and FreqSex, you will burn even more calories.

FreqSex

How frequently do people have sexual relations? In their study of the sexual behavior of males, Kinsey, Pomeroy and Martin found that the average (mean) frequency of total sexual outlet for the average, white, American male under thirty was 3.27 per week. But there was tremendous variation in the types and frequency of sexual activity. Marital intercourse might provide as little as 62% of the orgasms of certain groups of married males. One man had ejaculated only once in thirty years and another man had averaged thirty outlets per week for thirty years. The former had sex

45,000 times as often as the latter![2] In another study, women reported similar though smaller rates: by the age of thirty, women reported an average of 2.2 sexual activities per week, 1.5 by 40, 1.0 by 50 and 0.6 by 60.[3] Alex Comfort states that the average frequency of intercourse is two or three times per week, and David Reuben claims that "a man" who has intercourse more than once a week and less than twice a day is probably normal.[4] We believe that a "normal" rate of sexual activity is however often you engage in it, as long as you are satisfied and you do not consciously avoid it or seek it out to prove something. This ranges from a couple of times a year to a couple of times a day. However, the "normal" rate is not the rate necessary to lose weight.

A single act of sexual intercourse consumes 150 calories.[5] This is for one hour of sexual activity which is about right for most people. Some people take as little as two minutes and some take four or more hours. Thus, intercourse consumes more calories than playing golf[6] for an hour without using a golf cart (133 calories) and almost as much as roller skating for an hour (200 calories). Having intercourse is also equal to a ten-mile bicycle ride.[7] Thus, you can see that simply increasing the frequency of sexual activity can result in weight loss. Wouldn't you rather have sex than ride a bicycle, especially when it is wet and cold?

There is another way of looking at this: 150 is the number of calories contained in four and one-half cups of cauliflower, fifteen sour pickles, eighteen medium clams, a medium lamb or veal chop, eighteen raw oysters, a hot dog, one half of a roasted chicken breast, a couple of slices of bread, or two cups of vegetable soup. If you increase the frequency with which you have sex from two to eight times a month, you could eat an additional three more pieces of peach pie, three hundred bouillon cubes, six cups of potato chips, eighteen grapefruits, apples, or cups of sauerkraut, nine bananas, or fifty-four apricots. Thus, if you are already fit, Swell-Wimp enables you to eat more of your favorite foods without gaining weight.

Since one hour of sexual activity burns only 150 calories, Swell-Wimp results in slow weight loss which studies have shown is the best way. If you have intercourse twice a month, increasing the frequency to twice a week (eight times a month) will consume nine hundred additional calories. This is equal to playing cards for ten hours, throwing a Frisbee for five hours, playing seven and one-half hours of golf or standing around at cocktail parties for fifty hours. Again, which would you rather do?

Sex is Cheap and Convenient

We heartily agree with Alex Comfort when he says, "Sex is in fact the least tiring physical recreation for the amount of energy expended" (230). Also, keep in mind that SexAct is cheaper and easier than most other forms of exercise.[8] To golf, you must purchase clubs, pay fees and travel to the course. To cycle, you must buy a bike, mirror and helmet.[9] To play cards, you must round up four or more players, maybe travel to someone's home, and possibly lose substantial amounts of money and you probably will consume junk food and high-calorie beverages as you play. Clearly, sex is easier, cheaper and without a doubt more fun.[10]

Sex is also more convenient. You can have intercourse any time of day or night, but you cannot play golf at night. Weather has no effect on when you engage in *coitus exercisus*, but you cannot ride a bicycle in the snow (or you shouldn't) and it's dangerous to ride at night. SexAct isn't dependent upon the schedules of several other people; it's hard to round up your card-playing or basketball-playing partners on the spur of the moment.[11]

You are much more likely to have a better attitude about exercising if the form of exercise is SexEx. Sex feels good and makes you feel good. Pumping iron, chopping wood, doing calisthenics and so on are boring and tiring and it's hard to maintain a good attitude when you have to go out jogging in the rain and cold. As we pointed out earlier, your attitude is the most important factor in losing weight.

Mindless Useless Exercise

Incidentally, if you have the time, money, energy and need to engage in traditional exercises such as jogging, riding a stationary bicycle[12] or doing aerobics in front of the TV, then you have the time, money, energy and need to get off your duff and do something useful. Grab a garbage bag and pick up trash from along the highways and streets. We are pleased that in the last twenty-five years Americans have come to understand the importance of regular exercise. But, we are appalled that in such a short time it has become not only acceptable, but also common, for grown men and women to dress in expensive, garish exercise "outfits," don their Walkmans and hand weights and take to the streets and roads. Others, for whom sweatpants are stretch pants, jump up and down in front of the TV or *en masse* to the beat of high-energy music. Still others mount expensive pieces of equipment designed to simulate motions that the users can accomplish for free (walking, pedaling, stepping and so on) and then repeat the motions again and again until they work up a sweat, feeling, apparently, that they have accomplished something.[13] Have they (we) no shame? Does nothing strike us as ridiculous?

What has happened to us? Does it make sense to pay a kid to mow the lawn while we jog? Is it sensible to drive two blocks to purchase low-fat cookies and diet soda?[14] If so many of us have so much money for clothing and exercise equipment, why is there still hunger in this country? If so many of us can find time to attend to our own bodies, why are so many children failing in school? If you want to lose weight, then eat less or do more: help clean up your neighborhood or community, become an aide at your local school, volunteer at a nursing home or hospital, wash your own car, paint your own house, mow your own lawn. You can still wear your silly outfits while you do many of these things. It seems that there are plenty of people who have the time, money, and energy.

Former-president Bush, a man with money, energy and desire, had lots of time for exercise. How could this be? For many less-pampered people, there aren't enough hours in the day to get everything done. Where did he find the time to jog, play tennis and horseshoes, fish, hunt, and so on? President Clinton jogs and golfs. Shouldn't he, of all people, be extremely busy?[15] Shouldn't it be a given that when someone becomes President ("leader of the free world"), he or she forgoes vacations for the duration of his or her term? Vacations from what? The long drive to work? Stress from dealing with thirty kids in a classroom or meeting an impossible piece-rate? Repairing the leaking toilet and balky furnace? Relief from the noise the tenants upstairs make? Grocery shopping, washing clothes and feeding the kids? Working a second job to pay taxes, health-care premiums, the kids' tuition and the mortgage? It seems to me that two weeks in August (Congress is in recess) should be sufficient.

Maybe it is a case, as Ovid says, of *Parva leves capiunt animas.*[16] When was the last time that a President (or any politician) collapsed from overwork? After four years at a job, most people are lucky if they get two weeks of paid vacation. Am I the only one who finds it ridiculous for THE PRESIDENT OF THE UNITED STATES to take time away from the very pressing problems that face him to run around, going nowhere? Surely, there can't actually be times when he has nothing else to do! And the cost! I find it inconceivable that George Bush or any rational and caring individual could spend so much money (travel, Secret Service protection, etc.) so frequently for fishing, golfing and other vacations. If President Clinton were to engage in seasonal domestic tasks— mowing the White House lawn, shoveling snow, washing windows, painting the building, trimming the hedges, swabbing the portico and so on— he could stay on the White House grounds. Doing *useful* work instead of mindless exercise, he would serve as a model for the citizens of this country. Further, money would be saved: the number of maintenance workers and grounds keepers could be decreased and the enormous sums spent to transport him and provide protection every time he leaves the grounds would be reduced. At least when Ronald Reagan was president, he cleared brush at his ranch for exercise during vacations— not very interesting or mentally taxing, but useful.

It's probably too much to ask our pampered elite to actually do something useful when they exercise. But if our presidents, governors, legislators and other government officials were Swell-Wimpers, the country could save a substantial amount of money; we could close down most of the members-only spas and gymnasiums and sell off most of the exercise equipment. I urge you to write your Senators, Representatives, Council Persons, Mayors, etc.—your elected federal, state and local officials—and recommend Swell-Wimp to them. Lower your taxes![17]

More FreqSex

Simply put, FreqSex can help you lose weight. A recent study of prostitutes by Rrose Sélavy and Sheila Taque[18] found that almost all prostitutes (who engage in FreqSex, although not necessarily StrenSex) were within 3% of their ideal weight after factoring for drug use and disease.[19]

How often should you engage in FreqSex to lose weight? The simple answer is more frequently. Some of you have sex once a month and some of you have it everyday. If you increment from once a month to twice a month, you will burn additional calories, but not many and your weight loss over a year's time will be barely perceptible. If you increase to twice a day you will burn about nine thousand more calories a month and your weight loss will be dramatic, assuming that you also control your diet.

Burning more calories (more sex) and taking in more calories (eating more Twinkies) yields a net result of zero—no weight loss and no weight gain. Interestingly, this may be what some of you are looking for. You may be near your ideal weight, but frustrated because you cannot enjoy your favorite foods. Swell-Wimp (burning 150 calories) will enable you to eat more of what you like without gaining weight: one and one-half cups of boiled cabbage, a cantaloupe, thirty-six peanuts, a small serving of ice cream, a muffin, half a cup of berries, fifteen cups of celery, or a piece of chocolate cake. So, engage in SexAct as often as you and your partner like and can tolerate.

FreqSex Problems

However, FreqSex is not the best way to lose weight. One reason was hinted at in the last paragraph. A person can "take" just so much sex. There is always the possibility of injury.[20] The penis and vagina can become sore from overuse. You may injure various parts of your body; for example, the male's knees and elbows and the female's buttocks sometimes become abraded if the missionary position is always used. Of course, there is always the possibility of heart attack, heat stroke, and exhaustion.

The risk of injury can be reduced by slowly working up to maximum frequency over a period of weeks, allowing your bodies to adjust. This is especially important if you have been having sex infrequently. Varying positions and techniques (see Chapter 10) can also help. Extended foreplay (see Chapter 5) warms you up before each session. As with any physical exercise, you should be sure to cool down afterward (see Chapter 22). You must watch your diet closely, not only to monitor calorie intake, but also to supply your body with the things it needs to recuperate and repair damage.[21]

Most of us were told by our moms to wait an hour after eating before swimming, playing basketball and so on. We cannot definitively say that you should or should not wait after eating before engaging in SexEx. Usually, there is no need. After all, you will probably be lying down, and although your heart and respiration rates do increase and SexAct is an isotonic (as opposed to isometric) exercise, SexAct usually builds slowly to a peak. You should perform warm-up exercises and, of course, foreplay takes time also. Thus, there seems no real need to wait.[22] However, you risk cramping and injury if you immediately leave the table and begin SexAct (or even begin at the table).[23] Also, if you have some preexisting condition which requires that you exercise moderately, you should probably wait after eating so as not to put an extra burden on your system.

Another problem with FreqSex is that psychological injury may result, and certainly, the joy of spontaneity can be lost. This sort of thing sometimes happens to couples who want a baby but experience difficulty conceiving. Following their physician's orders, they have intercourse frequently, especially whenever there is even the remotest chance that the female is ovulating. Very soon "doing it" becomes a chore, something to be done, even if one partner has just worked a double shift. As time passes and they continue to fail to conceive, they become increasingly tense, which, unfortunately, decreases the chance that an egg will be fertilized. The same thing can happen when you are increasing the frequency of SexAct to lose weight. If you do not see results in a short time, you become frustrated and/or disillusioned. This causes sex to become even less enjoyable as you do it more and more frequently in order to burn calories. Ironically, the more you do it, the less you like it. This can be a major problem, especially if the two partners are not committed to Swell-Wimp to the same degree.[24]

Our advice is to engage in SexAct *quantum libet* (whenever you want). Be alert for signs that something is wrong or that you are not up to it and modify your timing and technique accordingly. There can be no doubt that increasing the frequency of SexAct can lead to substantial weight loss without injury if you heed the cautions we have just mentioned. Remember, *ne quid nimis*![25]

Chapter 4

StrenSex: More Strenuous Sexual Activity

"Vigorous sex is like a mini-workout," says Dr. Alfred Franger, Associate Professor of Obstetrics, Gynecology and Psychiatry at the Medical College of Wisconsin in Milwaukee.[1] Making sexual activity more strenuous is better than increasing the frequency of sexual activity; that is, StrenSex is better than FreqSex. First, you can increase the frequency only so much; eventually, your every minute will be devoted to foreplay, SexEx, postplay, eating and sleeping. However, you can almost always make your SexAct more strenuous. Remember, that more strenuous means burning more calories, not necessarily harder or more difficult. Second, having sex more frequently can be boring, but there are always additional, interesting ways to make sex more strenuous.[2] Although the same cautions from the last chapter about physical and psychological injury apply to StrenSex, our experience has been that you are more likely to achieve weight loss by increasing the strenuousness rather than the frequency of SexAct. In the following chapters we explore methods of modifying SexAct to become StrenSex; we discuss warm-up, foreplay, postplay, attire, techniques and positions, vocalization, strength, equipment and muscle control.

Over the last couple of decades we have been given much information about diet and exercise but it has had little effect. Malcolm Gladwell points out that in the 1960s 17% of middle-aged Americans met the clinical definition of obesity; in 1998 that figure had risen to 32%. The number of Americans who fall into what epidemiologists call Class Three Obesity (can't fit into an airline seat) has risen 350% in the last 30 years.[3] Why do we keep getting fatter? Because the media bombard us with silly, conflicting and partial information. Silly? Recently, our local evening news show did a report about the benefits of fencing for older people (every local station shows these canned "healthcasts" several times a week). The report couldn't have had relevance for more than five people in the entire audience! Frequently we are given the results of some study based on dubious premises, involving extremely small samples. Twenty-five years ago much of this information would have been considered preliminary or placed in its context as one small piece of a very large (nutritional) puzzle. Today, reports in obscure journals are reported widely as if they were the truth, the whole truth. More information is not synonymous with better information. People become confused (one day oats are good for the heart and the next day they are not). People switch to egg substitutes, having some vague notion that nutritional cholesterol is converted into serum cholesterol by the stomach (or liver or pancreas or kidneys) and dumped directly into the circulatory system which it immediately clogs up. Until the next week when it is reported that eggs are an excellent source of protein and we all need protein to maintain good health!

Further, advertisements for low-fat and reduced-calorie products and health foods are everywhere. Today we know more about nutrition but we know less about eating well. *Consumer Reports* advises that we should be careful with high-fat, high-calorie salad dressings; we should use no more than a tablespoon. Bosh! If you are eating a salad composed of tomatoes, lettuce, onions, cauliflower, carrots and other tasty and nutritious veggies, you simply don't have to worry whether you have put one or two tablespoons of salad dressing on it. There can't be more than five people in the entire United States who have avoided obesity by using low-calorie, low-fat salad dressing (and two of them guzzled it straight from the bottle). People hear what they want to hear and latch onto this or that tidbit from the gushing information stream. All people need to know is that they should beat a balanced diet and eat moderately. Common sense, but who wants to hear (or broadcast) that?

Malcolm says that three things affect a person's weight: diet, exercise and genetic inheritance. Like other animals, humans seem to have a predetermined setpoint, a weight that the body strives to maintain. You can diet and exercise but you can't change your genetic makeup, so reducing your weight below its setpoint is difficult. But there is some evidence that if you can keep the weight off for an extended period of time (2–3 years), you can establish a new lower setpoint. Because Swell-Wimp is a long-term method of weight reduction, it can help you do this. It requires no special diet, no special equipment. It's easy, it's natural and it's fun. Try it for a couple of years. What have you got to lose (except excess pounds)?

In Chapter 3 we said that one hour of sexual activity burns about 150 calories. The Women's Network at www.ivillage.com claims that one hour of "sex" burn 80+ calories per hour. We believe this figure is much too low. Von Kreisler, on the other hand, reports much higher figures: a 120-pound woman can burn up to eight calories a minute making love and a 180-pound man can burn up to twelve calories.[4] This computes to 480 calories per hour for women and 720 for men, far above our 150 calorie figure. We feel that few people maintain Von Kreisler's peak exertion rate for a full hour. We use a more conservative 150-calorie rate because we feel no need to "hype" Swell-Wimp.

However, many men and women do not expend even 150 calories when they engage in SexAct. Historically, women have been the passive partners in sexual intercourse. They did not expend much energy, just lying there.[5] There is no reason that women should be languid during sexual activity (even though women are generally less aggressive than men). It was once (mistakenly) thought that women did not enjoy sex (even disliked it!) and that they simply endured while the man "did the nasty" (and for months afterward if they became pregnant). This notion has been shown to be false and today women have much more liberated attitudes about sex.[6] Increasing the *frequency* of intercourse for a passive partner (male or female) will not result in the expenditure of many more additional calories. If he or she takes *a more active part* in the activity, even if not engaging in the activity more frequently, he or she will burn more calories. Both men and women can benefit from modifying their sexual practices to be more active, strenuous—to burn more calories.

It is helpful to view SexEx like any other exercise—a physical activity that burns calories (to lose or maintain weight) and improves fitness. As with other forms of exercise, you need long-term goals (I want to lose 20 pounds) and short term goals (I'm going to chop a cord of wood today). You need to watch your diet and keep some kind of records (recording the number of wieners eaten, blocks laid, balls hit, fees paid, etc.). And, of course, before beginning an exercise program you should get a physical examination.

Before beginning to chop wood or play tennis (or whatever), you should warm up. This loosens the muscles and tells the lungs and heart (and other organs) to start working harder. Next, you begin exercising slowly and build to peak caloric expenditure. This helps to avoid injury (for example, a "cold" muscle tears more easily). Finally, you cool down. Your body is operating at an accelerated rate and it needs to be slowly brought back to normal. Although a good exercise program does not require that you become obsessed with record keeping, warming up and cooling down, it is important to be systematic and attentive to detail, but this becomes second-nature quickly.[7]

Some of you are pretty lax about details[8] and will have to get your acts together (pun intended). Swell-Wimp (nor any other weight-loss and weight-maintenance program) simply will not work if you do not take it seriously, pay attention to details and exercise regularly.

If you have good intentions but are really deficient in will power, you may not be ready for Swell-Wimp which requires some self-motivation. You may need to try a program that cedes to others some of the responsibility for achieving weight loss. We would like to mention one such program (although we do not endorse it): The Fat Squad run by former Marine Sergeant Joe Bones. You sign a contract with The Fat Squad which allows the "calorie cops" to physically restrain you from breaking your diet (whether at home, work or a social function). Their motto is "You can hire us but you cannot fire us. Our commandoes take no bribes."[9] Hopefully, after working with The Fat Squad for a while you will find that you have gained the self-discipline to become a Swell-Wimper. Bones' progrm is extreme, but it may be the only solution for some. You can find out more about The Fat Squad by visiting www.joeyskaggs.com.

Those of you who are overly fastidious[10] will have to loosen up a little. You can be so concerned with record keeping and timing (seven minutes of foreplay, four minutes of postplay), that you cease to focus on the important thing: pleasurable, energy-intensive SexAct.

StrenSex is SexAct that is more strenuous than usual. "Usual" depends upon you. If you are a vigorous sexual athlete, then be more vigorous. If you're lethargic, then so something, anything. In the following chapters we will explain how to modify SexAct to become StrenSex; but here are two brief examples how anyone can increas the number of calories expended during SexAct. First, wear a coat. The additional weight will make you "work" harder and your body will also work harder trying to keep you cool. Second, chew gum (sugar-free, of course). Like fidigeting, chewing gum is not an energy-intensive activity, but every little bit helps especially if you do if for an extended period of time. Additionally, gum chewing can give a woman just a touch of adolescence or dumb blonde (especially if you "crack" the gum) and for men it can add a hint of Robert Redford. Be careful, of course, not to choke in the passion of climax.

Chapter 5

Warming Up and Foreplay

Warm-up and foreplay can help you to avoid injury, improve the quality of the primary sex act, and burn additional calories. In this chapter, we discuss foreplay and warming-up specific parts of the body before SexEx. In a later chapter, we discuss methods of strengthening some of these same body parts.

When we become sexually stimulated, a number of involuntary physiologic changes occur: there is an increase in adrenal and salivary secretions, pulse rate, blood pressure, peripheral circulation and nervous tension; blood flows into the eyes, lips, ear lobes, nipples, penis, clitoris, genital labia, vaginal walls and nose.

At climax, there is a sudden release which produces local spasms or more extensive and even all-consuming convulsions; control of the voluntary muscles is reduced. In men there are contractions of the rectal sphincter at .8-second intervals and ejaculation of semen. In women there are contractions of the uterus, vagina and rectal sphincter at .8-second intervals. Contractions of the abductors and adductors of the legs may cause them to move and twitch.[1] The toes curl,[2] the legs and arms bend or are rigid, the fingers curl, and the abdominal muscles contract. The intense feeling of orgasm lasts for only a couple of seconds (unfortunately)[3] and in women it is followed by vaginal contractions (many women don't distinguish between the two).[4] Although quite complicated, all of this happens without conscious involvement; a primitive part of the brain takes over (the pleasure as well as the pain center of the brain).

During orgasm, there is an involuntary arching of the back which drives the entire body forward, the heart rate can zoom to 160 or more and blood pressure can double. Clearly, your cardiovascular system should be in good shape or your sexual performance may suffer: the male may not be able to obtain or sustain an erection and the woman may pass out.[5] It is even possible that you might suffer serious injury, such as a heart attack.[6][7][8] Further, you can easily injure your back. Most people just don't realize how many back problems (one of the most common ailments in this country, and one that physicians can rarely do anything about) are due to involuntary thrusting by participants whose back muscles are weak (see Chapter 8 for more information). Thus, warming up for SexEx is very important.

Attitude

The proper attitude is necessary to get the most benefit from warm-up and foreplay. You are probably aware of the role of foreplay in erecting the penis[9] and lubricating the vagina, but you may not know that warming up before foreplay can help you avoid injury and improve performance. Although we use the word "performance" here, it should not be read with its traditional associations of role playing, either active or passive. An active role that men sometimes think they must play is being macho—able to satisfy any woman several times a day ("I'm hard. You ready?"). Another is that men may be insensitive ("Thanks for the sex. See ya baby."). Another is that men should be aggressive ("If you loved me you would.") and women reluctant ("If you loved me you wouldn't ask."). Another is that men may be stupid ("I don't need no stinking rubber."). Another...well, you get the idea. Sex is not an activity during which you actively play a part or passively assume a role. It is not something for which you should seek applause. Just be yourself; you may, in fact, be macho, aggressive, insensitive or stupid. If not, don't think that you have a duty to be something that you are not.[10] Further, performance anxiety can ruin sexual experience.

It has been known for centuries that females have the physical capability of experiencing two or more orgasms within a short time without dropping below the plateau level.[11] Continued sexual interest and stimulation often results in additional climaxes.[12] Interestingly, multiple orgasms occur more frequently during masturbation than intercourse because of the relative ease of continuing sexual stimulation and the lack of distraction due to concerns about the partner.[13] In fact, females have an almost unlimited orgasmic potential.[14] Although men cannot experience multiple orgasms (alas),[15] occasionally a partial or full erection may be maintained during the refractory period, but usually it subsides fully and completely. Some men achieve six or more full orgasms in a few hours if they aren't stressed and don't attempt it daily,[16] but most can't attain a second erection for quite a long time.[17]

Since the male has very little control of his penis (it is barely capable of independent movement) and limited orgasmic potential, it is crucial that he warm up those few muscles that give him some control. On the other hand, because the female has considerable control of her vaginal muscles and tremendous orgasmic potential, it is incumbent upon her to warm up them so as to be able to make extensive use of them during intercourse.[18]

Warm-Up Exercises

The first thing to do to warm up is to rub the important areas used during SexEx— the arms and legs, shoulders, genitalia, etc. This increases blood flow to these areas. Rubbing also feels good; unlike other forms of exercise, SexEx is pleasurable. Rubbing (especially of the sex organs) also increases sexual arousal.[19]

Females can warm up their vaginal muscles by doing Kegel exercises: tighten and release the muscles that control urination and defecation as if you were holding back both at the same time. You will feel a kind of internal lifting as the muscles tighten.[20] If you insert one or two fingers into the vagina while doing the exercises, you can feel it tighten. Kegel exercises can be performed sitting or standing and while doing other work.[21] The contractions should be held only for a few seconds and repeated ten or fifteen times to warm up the muscles. A woman should also warm up her thigh muscles by imagining there is something between them (or place something or someone between them) and tightening her thighs to squeeze it.

Males can warm up the muscles that enable them to move their penises by standing and tightening and releasing the muscles used to stop micturition. This draws the erect penis upward and then allows it to drop. It is interesting to ask why the muscles used to control elimination of bodily wastes are also the muscles that give us some control of our sexual organs. And why are the sexual genitalia so close to the rectum?[22] Why is the penis the conduit of both urine and sperm and why are the orifices of urination and impregnation so close together in women? It could be argued that women are evolutionarily superior to men because they have three orifices for sex, defecation and micturition while men have only two.[23] Primitive animals, such as birds and frogs, have only one (the cloaca); more advanced animals, including male humans, with more specialized body parts, have two; and the most advanced animals, female humans, have three.

In any case both males and females should also do some pelvic thrusts (to warm up the important back and groin muscles) and some tongue exercises; use the same exercises that are used to strengthen these areas, but only enough to warm up (see Chapter 8).

In addition to the penis and vagina, other areas need to be warmed up: the toes which support much of the top partner's weight; the shoulders and arms; the abdomen and small of the back (the most used muscles during intercourse); and the neck which most people ignore but is very important. Improper nuchal warm-up and weak and ill-controlled neck muscles can spoil a sexual event due to tiredness, lack of control and pain.

Pushups are excellent for warming up the shoulders, arms, back and toes simultaneously. Women who find pushups difficult can do half-pushups (supporting their weight on their knees instead of toes) and then do toe lifts (while standing, raise yourself up from your flat feet to tippy-toe).

Windmills (moving your arms like windmills) will also loosen the shoulders and back muscles and, if done fast enough and long enough, can increase heart and lung rates. Belly arches (lie on your belly and raise your head and feet off the floor toward the ceiling) are good for the back muscles. Head rolls (roll your head in a circle over your left shoulder, back, right shoulder and chest) loosen the neck muscles. Neck arches (lie on your back and raise your poop off the floor[24] by supporting your weight on the back of your head and your feet) warm up and strengthening the neck and shoulders.

There are several ways to increase your heart and respiration rates: jumping jacks (straddles), running in place and rapid toe-touching. We recommend that you avoid sit-ups because they are very tiring and an abdominal muscle can be torn if you do not roll upward properly. Also avoid deep knee-bends; they can damage the knees. Pull-ups offer nothing; you do not need big biceps.

If you have exercise equipment, you can use it to warm up. Our study subjects found that rowing machines and stationary bicycles are especially useful. Riding a stationary bicycle will loosen the legs and get the heart and lungs working. If it has reciprocating handlebars, the shoulders, back and arms will also be warmed up. In fact, if you do head rolls as you ride, you will take care of everything except the toes.[25] A rowing machine is also good; in fact, it exercises the back muscles even better than a bicycle. Again, you can do head rolls as you row and toe exercises afterward.[26] See Chapter 13 "Equipment" for more information.

Warming Up Naked

Warming up (and the exercises discussed in later chapters) should be done in a naked or nearly naked state. This allows the body to cool itself more easily and there are several important psychological benefits.[27] First, when you exercise naked, you feel that you are doing more work than if you were clothed. To test this out, undress and then wash the dishes or rake the lawn. You will find that you are more aware of each body part and its movement. This awareness gives you the feeling that you are doing more. Normally (clothed), we take the body's actions for granted. Second, naked exercise makes you feel lighter, freer, more nimble and graceful, because clothing no longer inhibits your movements and because, again, you are aware of your body's movements.

A third benefit is that naked exercise can be sexually arousing. You are aware of your naked body and feel that you are doing something slightly naughty (we are used to being naked only while bathing, not while taking out the garbage or vacuuming the rug). The movement of your body parts, freed of the restrictions of clothing, is enhanced. Now your breasts sway back and forth rhythmically while your inner upper-arms, speckled with perspiration, slide up and down gently caressing each breast in turn (the movement of the handlebars). Your inner thighs slide past each other on a film of moisture (peddling). Your penis or breasts tentatively descend toward the floor, gently touch the rug and retreat quickly, apprehensive, yet tantalized, about the next meeting (push-ups). As you run in place or do jumping jacks, you feel the brush of air as it passes through your crotch and about your external genitalia. The breasts, nipples erect and proud, exult in their freedom and scurry about first high, then low. The penis strikes the thigh with a satisfying slap and rebounds toward the other thigh, there to be rebuffed also.[28]

Naked warm-ups can be quite exciting, but you should NOT continue to sexual climax. Warming up involves work energy; calories are burned as muscles work. Naked warm-ups also involve sexual energy; the human body in the state of sexual arousal also expends calories (see Chapter 2).

Remember, though, that the purpose of warming up is to loosen muscles and to increase heart and breathing rates—that is, to prepare for physical (sexual) activity. Additionally, you increase your strength a little and develop your flexibility a bit. However, they are not an end in themselves. If you do them for too long or with too much intensity, you will tire yourself, which you do NOT want to do.

When you begin Swell-Wimp, you may feel a bit sore and stiff. This is normal. If you warm up naked (and we can think of no reason why you shouldn't), you may experience some chafing. If so, you can wear an appropriate piece of clothing (panties, shorts, socks) until it disappears (a few days at most). Then resume warming up naked. You may receive some chaffing for the chafing, but usually it will not appear a second time. If you experience ecchymosis, wear a jock-strap or bra for a few days until your body becomes used to the activity.

Warming-up can be done alone, but we recommend that partners do it together.[29] This is especially good in the earliest phase of warm-up when you rub each other's bodies. If you warm up alone, you must stroke your own penis or nuzzle your own nipples, which is usually less pleasurable. Also, you must use your hands (for the most part) to rub your body parts. When you warm up together, she can stroke the penis with her inner thighs and he can nuzzle her nipples with his penis.

Doing it together makes warm-up less boring; it allows each partner to keep an eye on the other insuring proper warm-up which will result in fewer injuries; it is sexually arousing; and it leads naturally into foreplay. In fact, although much of this book is devoted to instructions, often step-by-step, in a good sexual event each stage should blend seamlessly into the next—warm-up into foreplay, foreplay into primary sexual activity.

Foreplay

Because SexEx is EXERCISE, you must not omit warming up. Because SexEx is SEXUAL, foreplay must not be ignored. Foreplay takes you from partial to complete sexual arousal while expending energy. And it's fun![30]

Shere Hite says that foreplay is a strange term. She points out that it occurs before intercourse, but since women receive little clitoral stimulation during intercourse (most positions), for them it really isn't beFORE play. For males, stimulation of his partner's clitoris is part of foreplay, but it is the REAL play for women. When the real play begins for males (intercourse), stimulation usually subsides for most females (which may result in no play).[31] Hite is correct, and probably a better term than "foreplay" should be found. What frequently happens (especially if the partners are sensitive to each other's needs) is this: both partners' sexual arousal is heightened by foreplay; the woman is stimulated to non-coital orgasm; and the male achieves coital orgasm. Knowledgeable people admit that there is no need to strive for simultaneous coital orgasm.[32] If it happens, it's nice, but the attempt too frequently results in unilateral (male) climax. However, Hite fails to take into account the importance of foreplay in generally heightening sexual arousal for both males and females—showering, undressing, touching, kissing, etc. This is a time when much sexual energy is expended.

Foreplay is a natural part of SexAct. It includes any activity that involves sexual contact, is sexual in nature and precedes sexual intercourse. Different people do different things during foreplay and few people need instruction in this area. It includes stroking, nuzzling, rubbing, licking, caressing,[33] love talk (see Chapter 6), kissing,[34] and many other actions. Many men might be surprised to learn that the earlobes and the area behind the ears are erogenous zones and they may be kissed, nuzzled and bitten (gently).[35]

Kinsey provides information about what is useful during foreplay. In general, women are not as aroused by looking at live males (clothed or nude) as men are looking at live females. Women are also not as aroused by viewing opposite-sex genitalia.[36] Thus, slowly stripping and parading around is more arousing to men than women. Still, most of us are to some degree scopophiliacs and ecdysiasts so the placement of mirrors in the bedroom can be very stimulating.[37]

You may want to decorate the foreplay location (your bedroom, for example) with erotic visual materials to stimulate arousal and heighten the expenditure of sexual energy. Erotic prints and paintings make very nice additions to the bedroom walls.[38] But you should keep in mind that only 12% of females are aroused by seeing photographs, drawings, or paintings of nude figures, while 54% of males are. Thus, lying together and leafing through *Playboy* or *Playgirl* or watching yourselves in a ceiling mirror will probably be more beneficial to the man. Women are not as aroused as men by viewing burlesque shows or pornographic films. Women do respond to films containing erotic (as opposed to sexual) situations. Thus, a woman may find an R- or X-rated film more stimulating than a porno film.

Lighting is important: women prefer sexual activities in the dark while men prefer light, apparently because (as just mentioned) they are more susceptible to visual stimulation.[39] Thus, low lighting is a good compromise (candles are nice).

Music can help establish a mood (we discuss music at greater length in the next chapter). You should choose your foreplay music carefully. For example, although the group "Foreplay" plays excellent jazz, the tempo is probably too fast and the rhythm too irregular for good foreplay.[40] During foreplay you will want music that is arousing, even romantic. On Saturday night 20 March 1999 the British Classical FM station played "music to make love by"; couples who conceived on that night would

have children born at the dawn of the new millenium. Among the selections broadcast were: *Chi bel sogno di Doretta* by Puccini; the aria "Hueten Moch" from Bach's
Coffee Cantata (BWV 211); Ravel's *Bolero*; the 2nd movement of Bach's *Suite #3 in
D Major* ("Air on the G String"); the Intermezzo from Mascagni's *Cavalleria
Rusticana*; and Saint-Saens *Symphony No. 3 in C*. We are not suggesting that you
should conceive a child, but the press release described these musical pieces as very
stimulating (we are not familiar with any of them) so you might want to try them.[41]

Swell-Wimp foreplay differs somewhat from the non-Swell-Wimp variety. Since
you and your partner have already decided to engage in SexEx and have warmed up,
the aim of foreplay is not to determine if your partner wants to "get it on." Swell-
Wimp foreplay is not tentative; your partner will not reject your advances and you are
both at least partly aroused. Thus, your primary (if not only) aim is to bring yourselves to complete arousal.

Teasing during foreplay expends many calories. For example, one partner can
tease the other's penis to erection. Next, the penis is allowed to return to the detumescent state. Then that partner can stimulate his partner until her labia become engorged
and her nipples erect. While she cools down, she again stimulates her partner. This
sort of teasing can expend MUCH energy. As always, do not overdo it; too much teasing can result in tiredness and frustration.

Incidentally, teasing can be used to burn calories while one partner is asleep
(assuming you sleep with your Swell-Wimp partner). This causes him or her to burn
some calories through sexual arousal. You burn some calories due to sexual arousal
and activity and it gives you something better to do than count sheep.[42] With practice,
you can become proficient enough to arouse your partner without awakening him or
her. But if he or she becomes sufficiently aroused, you should be willing to engage in
SexEx (it would be mean to tease only). And if he or she doesn't want to be bothered,
you should stop without feeling resentment. Of course, you should inform your partner that you may tease during the night; otherwise, if he or she wakes and finds you
playing with his or her body, he or she may wonder what you are doing and why.

There is another reason that it is important to tell your partner that you may tease
during the night. When we wake up, there is a brief time during which we are not
asleep and not awake. Some of us awaken pleasantly and some of us awaken grumpi-
ly, even violently. When your partner wakes, he or she might strike out and you could
be injured. You should understand that even the nicest people can act unpredictably
when awakened. Some courts have even ruled that we are not responsible for our
actions during this time. Usually, the teasing is incorporated into the sleeping person's
dream and he or she awakens gradually and in a good mood. But in the dream the

sleeper might be resenting the teasing and strike out when he or she awakens. Thus, you could be punched, slapped or kicked; most people when they wake up do not grab things (the clock or water glass from the night table or a shoe from the floor) before striking out. You should not react by striking back (or by taking your partner to court). Thus, a positive thing (teasing) could become a negative thing (it ruins a sexual relationship). All things considered, you should probably not tease your partners while they sleep unless you are 99% sure they will awaken calmly.

Dancing

Dancing can be done during warm-up or foreplay. Contact dancing can be very erotic. This is one of the reasons that some religions prohibit it, whether waltzing, jitterbugging or tangoing.[43] We would add that it is especially arousing if done naked.[44] Dancing expends energy and can be done moderately or vigorously. Even if done with clothes on, it can be arousing. You can stroke your partner and touch those spots that arouse your partner and yourself. You can also strip as you dance. Naked touch-dancing heightens visual and tactile stimulation. If you dance vigorously, you may want to wear a bra or jock strap in order to maintain your rhythm and prevent bruising.

How Long?

Kinsey reports that in 11% of marriages, foreplay is limited to three minutes or less; in 22%, it extends to twenty or more.[45] Three things should be noted about these figures. First, they are limited to married couples.[46] Second, the figures are from a time when only vaginal orgasm was thought to be "normal"; a woman who could achieve only non-vaginal, clitoral orgasms was called "frigid."[47] Thus, males generally spent less time stimulating their partners during the pre-intercourse period and went directly to intercourse when it became apparent that the female was "close to coming."[48] Third, none of the subjects that Kinsey interviewed were engaged in Swell-Wimp; they were not trying to maximize their energy expenditure during SexAct. Therefore, it seems to us that (generally speaking) most couples today spend more time in pre-coital activities (foreplay). Still, this does not answer the question "How long should warm-up and foreplay take?" We do not want to avoid answering the question, but it depends. You don't want to spend so much time in warming up and foreplay that you lose interest, or become exhausted, or begin to sweat profusely or even overheat! How much time do you normally spend? Then longer. The more time you spend in warming up and foreplay, the more calories you burn up!

Even if you go on to intercourse from foreplay, the female may, of course, climax during foreplay and the male can climax without intercourse. Most of the activities and techniques that we discuss in the following chapters are also applicable to foreplay. The aim is to expend as many calories as possible without going to extremes. Remember, Swell-Wimp is supposed to be EASY, natural and fun.

Chapter 6

Vocalization and Erotolalia[1]

In the last couple of chapters, we have explained the differences between FreqSex and StrenSex, pointing out that FreqSex can take you only so far toward fitness; StrenSex is to be preferred for a serious, long-term Swell-Wimp. We have discussed the importance of physically warming and the advantages of sexual foreplay. Now it is time to suggest specific ways that you can make SexAct into StrenSex.

How do you burn more calories during StrenSex? First, you could do things "harder"; that is expend more calories while doing the same things you always do. This is not easy because most things that you can do arduously become less pleasurable (hugging, kissing, and sucking). The female can squeeze her thighs firmly, but the male should not thrust severely (it will be less pleasurable for him and her). Thus, "harder" is not the way to expend more calories.

Better than "harder" is "more": almost anything EXTRA that you do will burn more calories. For example, if you were to lift dumb bells during SexEx, you would certainly expend a lot of energy. However, it wouldn't be easy or much fun. There are several convenient and interesting way to achieve StrenSex. In later chapters we will discuss dressing for Swell-Wimp and calisthenics-type exercises. In this chapter we cover vocalization.

Vocalization

Little attention has been given to the importance of vocalizing during SexAct.[2] Some people don't speak at all during SexAct, but *cum tacent clament* (their silence cries out); the fact that *magis mutus quam picis*[3] is not a case of *qui tacet consentit*.[4]

They have/need to speak: there may be some things[5] they should "get off their chests."[6] Most people speak some (love talk or comments such as "Your elbow is poking me") and many say much, but such vocalization is usually random, not consciously organized for a purpose. Talking, like any other activity, expends energy, and the proper and controlled expenditure of energy during SexAct is the topic of this book. Vocalization, which in a very broad sense includes articulate and inarticulate speech, cooing, singing, grunting, reciting poetry,[7] humming, whistling, laughing, crying, screaming, and so on, should not be overlooked when striving for StrenSex. Vocalization involves the lungs (diaphragm and associated chest muscles), abdominal muscles, neck and cheek muscles, tongue, and other structures. There is great opportunity here for energy expenditure.

If maximum energy expenditure is the aim, then stenorian is better than quiet, a lot is better than a little, and fast is better than slow; so quickly making a lot of loud noises expends the maximum amount of energy. Further, vocalizations that require lots of breath (diaphragm and chest movement), such as screaming and yelling are to be preferred. High tones (screaming and squeaking) require more energy. Low tones (moaning and grunting) require less effort, and it is easier to do more of them and to do them automatically. Thus, when you first add vocalization to your SexAct, you probably will find it easier to moan and grunt. When you become more proficient, you can switch to high-pitched sounds, like chirping and squeaking.

There are also psychological benefits to vocalization during SexAct. Many people, who are a bit inhibited about vocalization during sexual activity (especially men who are afraid of *lapsus linguae*[8]), are delighted to find that it is not very hard to abandon themselves wholeheartedly, and that eructed foque is fun. Any vocalization is better than none (in terms of energy expenditure), but organized vocalization is best. Throwing off inhibitions is good, but random, spontaneous vocalization is not very efficient. Further, *cacoëthes loquendi* (compulsive talking) and logorrhea[9] can be unpleasant for the listening partner. There are several types of efficient vocalization appropriate to Swell-Wimp, including running commentary, counting, mantras, singing and laughing.

Sex on TV, in the Movies and in Books

This is a good place to digress a bit and point out that violent and passionate SexAct as depicted on TV, in the movies and books is not the norm. Few people actually tear each other's clothes off (especially with their lips locked in a prolonged kiss) or roll off the bed and across the room while remaining coupled. Few men throw their partners onto a bed and most women do not dig their nails into their partner's body.[10] All of this makes for exciting and arousing drama, but it is not reality. Thus, you should not think that your sex drive is sub-normal because you don't do (or want to do) these things.[11] You should be yourself and do what is right for you, not what television, cinema, books or other people say you should do.[12]

People are individuals. Television, books, and cinema (popular not serious art) treat individuals as stereotypes (buffoonish husband, suave lover, self-effacing hero) or as members of classes (poor blacks, crooked cops, Latin lovers, victimized women, Italian mobsters). Subtlety is not the forte of TV and films. We are not sociologists and our purpose is not to write a sociological tract,[13] but we do want to urge you to see yourself as an individual interacting with other individuals. Do not take your cues from television, the movies, and books. Aggressive SexAct is not the norm nor is it right. Neither, however, is it abnormal or wrong. It is right and normal for some people.[14] If you and your partner(s) are among those people, then it is right and normal for you.[15]

So doing "harder" is not the way to expend more calories during SexEx. Doing more is better and vocalizing is an easy, convenient and interesting way to achieve StrenSex.

Running Commentary

A useful vocalization is the running commentary or critique, during which the partners continually remark on how they are feeling, what they are doing, what their partner is doing, how their partner is feeling, and so on. Although this is a bit pedestrian, it should not be shunned, especially if you have become accustomed to it, or if there seems to be a need for it because of dissatisfaction or insecurity on the part of one partner. Of course, if one partner's running commentary is consistently unfavorable, the other partner may be negatively affected.[16] Most of us don't like to be told again and again that we are pushing too hard, putting our tongues in the wrong places, going too quickly (or slowly), or leaning on the partner's hair or that we are too heavy or have cold hands. What your partner says during orgasm should never be used against him or her. So it might be useful if you and your partner agree to make only positive comments (when appropriate) during SexAct and hold negative comments until later. It is better to engage in neutral ("I'm going to raise my legs. I'm getting closer. That doesn't feel bad. I'm going to come. I'm going to come.") than negative commentary. Still, afterward you should let your partner know about anything unpleasant. It is not good, for example, for a woman not to tell her partner that he hurt her when he entered. There is no pleasure or honor in suffering silently. And positive feedback ("That's good. Do that again. I like it when you move your tongue back and forth like that.") can do wonders for your sex life.

Counting

Counting each caress, rub, thrust, and so on expends some energy and can become an unconscious activity. Keep in mind, however, that counting should not become part of an evaluative process. For example, "Three thrusts and you came. Where's the pleasure for me?" or "I rubbed your clitoris 178 times. I was too tired to wait any longer." You must resist the urge, should a given sexual episode be less than satisfactory, to use the counts against your partner.

Mantras

For those who find it difficult to concentrate on too many things at once, we recommend what we call a "sex-mantra." Like a mantra used during meditation, the sex-mantra is repeated over and over. Whereas during meditation the aim is to focus on the mantra and to clear the mind, the importance of the sex-mantra is to be able to engage in vocal exercise without having to concentrate on that very thing. We recommend that each person develop his or her own personal mantra and that partners experiment (your partner may hate your mantra). It is probably best to build from simple, easy sex-mantras monotonally repeated, such as "Oh my! Oh my!" to more complex ones, such as "I love Bosco; that's the drink for me." At first, any well-known, easily repeated phrase will do: "Oy vey," "Ya, sure," "Up yours," and "I was gonna say."

If you are up to it, you may want to try Latin vocalizations; the foreign sounds add a touch of the exotic and many Latin phrases are rhythmical, even musical: *nolens volens; una voce; stans pede in uno; suum cuique pulchrum;* or *uti non abuti.*[17]

Singing

Sex-mantras often develop into singing, which is a very good form of vocalization. The rhythm of songs can aid in ordering and timing your sexual events; for example, two stanzas of "Zippity Do Dah" during foreplay, enter on the chorus, repeat the chorus three times and finish with a reprise of the first stanza. Physical movements (such as pelvic thrusts) can be enhanced by the tempo of the song you sing: warm up to "Eve of Destruction" or "The Unicorn"; foreplay to "Lay, Lady, Lay"; primary activity accompanied by "Bang, Bang" and climax to the final stanzas of "Little Nash Rambler."

Humans have a natural instinct to favor rhythm. When a couple sings together, their physical movements become synchronized. For example, a duet of "Don't you know/ that's the sound of the men/ working on the chain/ gang...All day long they're singing/ Uh, uh/ Ah, ah" is perfect for coitus in most positions.

Singing makes us happy.[18] When a couple sings together, each feels happy. And they feel even happier as a couple doing two pleasurable things. Also, singing certain songs can result in double entendres[19] which can cause laughter or just make the activity more enjoyable. For example, the song "Working in the coal mines, going down, down, down" is wonderfully suggestive. You can also change the words of some songs (whose melody or rhythm you like) to be more suggestive.[20]

As you become more proficient at singing and SexAct, you can add more difficult material to your repertoire, including songs with alternating parts, such as "Let's call the whole thing off,"[21] "Ah, yes I remember it well"[22] and rounds like "Row, row, row your boat"[23] and "Frère Jacques."[24]

However, you should choose your songs carefully. Dr. Harold Zulo, of Columbia University, analyzed top-forty songs and *Time* covers from 1955 to 1989 and found that they predicted economic down-turns a year or more ahead of time.[25] There are two possible explanations for this: (1) people knew a year in advance that hard times were coming and reflected this knowledge in their choice of songs; (2) the songs that people sing contribute to the general attitudinal ether that all of us are immersed in and which affects us all, including our economic decisions; a negative ether results in choices which have a negative effect on the economy. If the second explanation is true, then choose your songs carefully, because you may contribute to a downturn in the economy especially since you will be singing them repeatedly.

There are other reasons for choosing your songs carefully. The rhythm of "El Toreador" (from Bizet's *Carmen*) is inappropriate for any sexual activity and will spoil the experience. Songs like "Modern Major General" are much too fast. Others, such as "My Buddy," "London Derrière"[26] and "Feelings," are much too slow except for the aged and infirm. If you have parrots or mynah birds near where you engage in Swell-Wimp, you should be careful about what you sing and everything else you vocalize because it may be repeated at your next dinner party.[27]

Here are some more songs you can choose from: Ain't She Sweet; Come and Play With Me; Blow the Man Down; Baby, Ain't It Hard?; Damnit Janet; Tighten Up; The Ballad of Sally in Our Alley; Blowin' in the Wind; Macho Man; Giddy-Up Go; Like a Virgin; Biological Time Bomb; Deep Within You; Love For Sale; and Don't Fence Me In.[28]

Laughter

Laughing is an excellent form of vocalization, but it is usually a spontaneous, unconscious activity. Still, you can place funny items around your SexEx location. *Playboy* and *The New Yorker* are excellent sources of cartoons (although the latter are a bit cerebral sometimes). You can use a photocopier to enlarge them. Funny posters and calendars are good too.[29] Photographs, ceramics, sculpture—anything that makes you laugh is suitable.

You can also play comedy albums, tapes and CDs. You should not worry that your attention will wander. Cyclic arousal, which we mentioned earlier in connection with teasing, means repeatedly becoming aroused and cooling down without orgasm. This burns calories and prolongs pleasure. It can cause no harm to your sexual organs, so enjoy it.[30] You can also memorize and repeat your favorite jokes. This works best during foreplay and postplay.

Laughter and giggling can be induced by tickling, either in especially sensitive spots, such as the feet, ribs and crotch, or anywhere on the body by the judicious use of a device such as a feather.[31]

Laughter is psychologically beneficial to both partners[32] and an excellent way to expend energy. Even a "philosophical [silent] laugh" burns some calories.[33] However, laughter is not usually rhythmical and, therefore, can interfere with physical rhythms. Thus, it is probably best to restrict its use to foreplay and postplay.

There can be no doubt that communication or lack of it between (among) sexual participants is important.[34] And, therefore, erotolalia can play an important role in SexAct. In a study by Dr. Paul Gillette 90% of the couples interviewed said that "sex talk" aroused them and 70% said that they did it regularly. The most arousing word is the F word followed by "cock," "cunt"[35] and "suck"—often repeated randomly without context. Others found oral fantasizing arousing (sometimes accompanied by acting out the fantasy).[36]

We Can't Do Everything Well

Although you may want to lose weight, gain muscle tone, and maximize pleasure, you cannot do everything at once. You cannot chant a sex mantra, sing and laugh at the same time. Trying to do too much can result in frustration since you are bound to fail at something. Remember that Swell-Wimp is supposed to be easy, natural and FUN. Frequently, when you engage in Swell-Wimp, you will want to proceed to the point of climax and stop. If you are trying to concentrate on too many things, you may pass the point of climax without being able to stop.[37] Orgasm is probably the most pleasurable aspect of sexual exercise and it burns a lot of calories. Keep in mind that at the point of climax, you lose almost complete control of yourself. As Emily Dickinson says in Poem 390, "It's coming—the postponeless Creature." Like vomiting, it is almost impossible to stop once you begin. Think of it as ascending one side a playground slide and descending the other. The climb up can be very pleasant but the trip down is more fun. Once you have reached the top and have begun to slide down, you cannot stop without extreme effort and possible injury.[38] When climaxing, conscious intentions count for little.

So be aware that no matter how you structure your sexual exercise, there comes a point that you must travel beyond. If you do not want to climax (it is the wrong time or you are in the wrong place), avoid reaching this point.[39] You **may want** to engage in forceful vocalization or shake your head from side to side or kick your legs up and down (to expend many calories), but you **will do** what your body wants. Do not become frustrated. Since you are unlikely to do anything that will increase your weight or reduce your state of fitness (eat a Ring Ding or drink a milkshake), go with it. It's nice to let go sometimes.

Thus, you should choose one type of vocalization and do it well or progress from one to another. We suggest small talk during foreplay. Then begin singing or chanting as coitus begins. At the appropriate stage, begin yelling or moaning. During postplay, engage in laughter, small talk, or singing (whatever seems right).

Most people deliberately or unconsciously speak during SexAct, often saying meaningless or even stupid things. However, as lawyers say, *cave quid dicis, quando, et cui*.[40] Isn't it better to divert the natural instinct to make noise during SexAct into a more productive channel? Try some of our suggestions and you will be amazed at how much more quickly you lose weight *con strepito*![41]

Chapter **7**

Dressing for Swell-Wimp

Kinsey reports that 90% of males with college-level education regularly engage in nude coitus, 66% with high-school level and 43% with grade-school level. Also 41% of college level males frequently sleep nude, 34% of high-school level and only 16% of grade-school level. Thus, the level of education achieved in part determines attitude toward nude coitus and nude sleeping.[1] He also reports that 67% of the older generation engage in nude coitus whereas 92% of the younger group do. Further, 37% of the older group sleeps nude, but 59% of the younger. Thus, the generation you were born into partially determines your attitudes toward nude coitus and nude sleeping.[2] It may seem unusual to have a chapter about dressing in this book; after all, as you can see, most people remove their clothing for SexAct. However, you can enhance sexual pleasure and increase the number of calories expended by carefully selecting a wardrobe.[3] It is well known that various "garments"—for example, frilly lace underwear, leather jock straps, clear plastic wrap—can be sexually arousing and you should include some of these in your wardrobe. If you feel sexy, you project sex appeal; if you feel like a lump, you project lumpy. Thus, you need to feel good to make your partner(s) feel good.[4]

Why Dress?

There are a number of reasons to incorporate a particular item in your SexEx wardrobe. First, if it pleases you and your partner and puts you in a good mood, you may want to include it. Such a garment may highlight one of your attractive or sexy features, have good memories associated with it or simply be "smart." However, you have to be practical. It may take too long to put on the evening gown your partner likes to see you in. And it may be impractical to don a complete set of scuba gear, even though your partner thinks you look macho in it.[5]

Second, an item may sexually arouse you or your partner. Again, you have to be practical. A pair of tight jeans, a muscle shirt, a thong-cut bathing suit, sweat bands, a baseball cap, boxing gloves—any of these are easy to put on and keep at hand. But it just may take too long to put on (and take off) a three-piece suit even though your partner says you look like ExecuStud. And some items, even though they are tremendously stimulating, may be inappropriate and even dangerous—for example, skis and skates. Of course, this depends upon your skill and familiarity with the items. Wearing a carpenter's tool belt or sequin studded leotards during SexEx would be too dangerous for most people, but maybe not for you. But, even if you are quite agile, you must be careful because in the heat of passion we often fail to be cautious. For example, if you decide to wear heavy footwear to add weight in order to burn more calories, you probably should not choose ice skates (you could break an ankle or lacerate your partner) or roller blades (you might careen around the room) unless you are an accomplished skater. Be careful and be moderate.

Third, you may want to include items that can contribute to weight loss. There are twenty-four square feet of skin on the average human body through which body heat is lost. Items made from close-weaved fabrics do not "breathe" and thus keep the heat in and cause you to sweat (which helps you to lose weight). So, nylon jackets, shirts, pants, and stockings are good as are items such as snowmobile suits, a Shadwell mantle and diving wet-suits, which are designed to keep the body's heat from escaping.[6] Simply wrapping a body part (the thighs or abdomen, for example) in plastic wrap during warm up can be beneficial. Garbage bags in various sizes are very useful.[7] You can put each leg into a full-sized garbage bag and use a garter or rubber band to hold them up. Smaller bags can be used for the arms. Large bags can be wrapped around the abdomen or buttocks and fastened with belts or string.[8]

Dressing to Burn Calories

Other items of this third category are those that cause you to work harder, primarily because they are heavy. Jeans are always good; they are somewhat heavy and comfortable to wear. Unfortunately, modern advances in fabrics have resulted in very light clothing (especially winter wear). A Woolrich hunting coat (red plaid wool) or

Pea coat (blue wool), especially if wet, is heavy and thus will help you to burn more calories than a modern ski jacket. Additional clothing can add weight, so you might want to try wearing several shirts, socks, panties or undershorts.[9] Or you can increase the weight of your current SexEx wardrobe by adding ornaments and decorations such as shoulder-knots, gold lace, colored satin, silver fringe and embroidery. Wear as much clothing as you want, as long as it doesn't get in the way of sexual pleasure or cause injury or overheating.

Moving additional weight during SexEx, of course, burns calories, so you might add to your "wardrobe" heavy things that can be worn, such as ankle and wrist weights, weighted bedroom slippers, heavy shoes, a diver's weight belt, a carpenter's tool belt, a football helmet, a baseball catcher's chest pad and so on. If you can manage the weight, and it doesn't turn you off or interfere with the pleasures of SexAct, then consider wearing it.

You can also modify some items of your regular wardrobe to meet the special needs of Swell-Wimp. For example, replacing buttons and zippers with Velcro enables you to begin exercising much more quickly (especially important if your schedule forces you to exercise where and when you can). Velcro can make garments that you or your partner find stimulating but too time-consuming to don, faster and easier to put on. For example, tight leotards or eight-button vests go on and come off more easily when Velcro is used. (You must be careful with Velcro, though: it will "stick" to hair and can be very painful to untangle.)

Do not overlook the usefulness of headwear. Humans can lose up to one-half of their body heat through their heads which is why we wear hats in the winter. Wearing one or more hats or babushkas during SexEx can keep heat in and, thus, cause you to perspire more quickly and more profusely. Diaphoresis is an indication that the body is working harder to keep cool and that calories are being burned. The best headwear for this purpose are knitted caps, such as watch caps and ski caps. They are warm, inexpensive, easy to put on and take off and unobtrusive.[10] Of course, you should remove the headwear if you become overheated.

You should take into account where you need to lose weight as you assemble your Swell-Wimp wardrobe. Since most people find being naked stimulating, you probably do not want to wear any more clothing than is necessary. Thus, you might wear a cap and two sweatshirts only (if you are heavy in the upper body) or a cap, and several pairs of stockings (if you are heavy in the legs). Of course, during warmup (and even foreplay and postplay) you should wear as much clothing as you like.

If you really, really like naked SexEx and would prefer not to wear any clothing, consider jewelry. Anything you wear adds weight that has to be moved as you exercise. Jewelry looks very nice set against the naked body and the body looks good tastefully adorned with jewelry. You can don extra earrings, necklaces, rings, wrist and ankle bracelets, or waist chains—each adds some weight. Wearing two Rolexes instead of one will significantly increase your caloric expenditure. Gold is heavier than silver and real pearls are heavier than ersatz. However, be cautious. Diamonds and other gems can lacerate your partner and it is easy for hair to become entangled in bracelets, necklaces and watch bands.

Footwear adds weight and thus causes you to burn calories. Many people are aroused by boots, especially thigh-high and leather boots. You can wear any kind (work, riding, knee, ski, hip, motorcycle, cowboy), but be sure they do not have buckles, studs, spurs or anything that can cause injury or put tape over the sharp edges. Choose footwear that you like, that turns you on and that is appropriate for your personality: bunny slippers, wing tips, saddle shoes, go-go boots, shower sandals or whatever.

Generally, footwear should be easy to remove so you can wear it for warmup and foreplay and remove it for intercourse.[11] Removing boots (for example) or exchanging them can be a part of foreplay.

The Importance of Hair

Most people do not think of hair as attire, but as we do with clothing, we choose our hairstyles, often matching them to an occasion (such as SexAct). We are not the first to point out the importance of hair in relation to SexAct; Vatsyayana discusses hair braiding, dressing hair with unguents and perfumes, and shampooing (which can be a very sensual and even erotic experience).[12]

Head hair has always been related to well-being and vitality. Especially in primitive[13] societies (but not only), it can reveal a person's well-being; a sick person's hair may fall out or be tangled and matted. Just as poverty or illness can show that the gods are displeased with you, unattractive hair indicates that you are physically or morally ill. As diet and health care improved, this linkage between physical health, attractiveness and moral standing weakened, but not completely. The presence of hair salons, barbers and hair dressers in hospitals is not just a sop to patients' vanities. Frequently, the first thing people want after surgery or an illness, is to "do" their hair. The hospital staff encourages this because attitude plays a large role in recovery. If patients want to look good (get their hair done), they are more likely to want to feel good (get well).[14]

Further, hair is seen as an indicator of a person's vitality and sexuality.[15] Remember Samson, whose strength and vigor lay in his hair?[16] And isn't it assumed that blonds/blondes have more fun? What constitutes sexy hair differs among societies. Some prefer long, loose hair. Others like greased hair. Some shave various regions of the head. Thus, greasy hair could indicate sickness or well-being, depending upon the society. But every society has some customs and traditions concerning hair "style" and hair care. Today, the limitations imposed by nature no longer restrict us as they once did. If our hair is the wrong color, or too thin or too curly or whatever, we can get it fixed by a trained hairdresser.

Hair has always contributed to sexual attractiveness. Medieval literature is full of puns about hunting the hare/hair (pubic).[17] Remember Belinda in Alexander Pope's *Rape of the Lock*?[18] Her hair is a symbol of her chastity as well as sexual allure and the theft of one of her locks by the Baron constitutes a kind of rape. Authors often use hair as a sexual symbol and a touchstone to a character's character. In Ibsen's play, *Hedda Gabler*, Hedda has thin auburn hair, but Thea, the character who represents freedom, vitality, and love, has abundant, wavy flaxen hair.[19] Interestingly, authors have concentrated almost entirely upon head hair.[20] Only recently have they described pubic hair, and never do they use it metaphorically and symbolically.[21] And hair is, of course, important in popular culture.[22]

Thus, you should give your head hair thoughtful consideration.[23] The style—pigtails, bouffant, crew cut, page boy, Mohawk, shoulder length—doesn't matter; choose what you and your partner like. Attractive hair will aid in arousing your partner. And as we have pointed out, sexual energy output alone can be considerable; if he or she is "turned on," your partner will use more energy. And if you like the way you look, you will feel sexier, and exude more sexual energy.

Cutting your hair does not affect its rate of growth, so it takes no more or less energy to grow long or short hair.[24] We do recommend that the hair style you choose not take too long to prepare. Although you can expend many calories preparing your coiffure, it may take so long that you (or your partner) no longer want to engage in SexAct. Also, your hairdo should be somewhat durable. If it is so delicate that it comes "undone" after a few minutes of sexual activity, it may have the opposite of the desired effect; it may become a "turn off."

Shaving

In Chapter 2 we said you should not shave head or body hair to increase performance as swimmers do. However, decorative shaving can enhance SexEx and even
revitalize a weak relationship. Today, head shaving (even by women) is not considered to be an extreme action as it once was.[25] In recent times, Alopecia has been considered sexy: the following are frequently named when people are asked whom they
consider sexy: Burt Reynolds, Telly Savalis, Bud Greenberg, Daddy Warbucks,
Patrick Stewart, Nikita Kruschev, Otto Preminger, Yul Brenner, Hank Snow, Dom
DeLuise, Michael Jordan, Willard Scott, Mikhail Gorbachev, Elton John, Irving
Lazar, Phil Collins, Charles Dutton, Kareem Abdul Jabar, Dolly Parton and Phyllis
Diller. Still, shaving your head may be more than you are willing to do.

However, shaving your pubic hair may result in a self-consciousness that can
enhance sexual activity just as wearing sexy underclothing can make you feel more
sexy (because YOU know that you are wearing a see-through bra or crotch-split
panties or no underwear at all[26]). When you feel sexy, you ARE sexy and others pick
up on it. Unlike when you shave your head, no one but you and your sexual partner(s)
will know you have shaved your crotch. Completely removing pubic hair (*crotchibus
in naturalibus*) can result in a pre-pubescent look, that many find very sexy. Shaping
pubic hair to spell a partner's initials or to look like a heart or wings or a downward
pointing arrow is easy and alluring.[27]

Males who usually shave their faces may want to let their beards grow. A couple-
of-days growth—the *Miami Vice* look—is now considered sexy. Allowing your beard
to grow can revitalize a relationship; you look more or less like a different person to
your partner and this injection of newness may be beneficial. Ask your partner what
she likes. You may be surprised to find that she is turned on by the Lenin, Fu Manchu,
Bowery bum or Elvis look. Shaving off a grey beard may make you look younger and
allowing your beard to grow may make you look more distinguished. Experiment.[28]

Shaving other body hair can also be sexually stimulating. When a male shaves his
legs, it can be very exciting for both him and his partner. She will feel his bare,
smooth legs for the first time, and he will feel bare skin against bare skin in places
and in ways he has never experienced before. Caressing her entire body with his legs
will be a new and very arousing experience for both. The same is true if the male
shaves his buttocks and performs *assinus asinum fricat* (heinie rubbing).[29] Once the
hair on the female leg is allowed to grow, it is usually soft and fine.[30] Of course, a
person who shaves her or his leg, pubic and armpit hair may feel colder.

Women can let some of their body hair grow to good effect. Some of you may be surprised to learn that not all women shave their underarm hair and that those who do not are not all low-class or from Eastern European countries and that female underarm shaving did not become widespread until recently.[31] If you don't shave your underarms, try it. You and your partner will appreciate the smoothness. If you do, try letting the hair grow. You and your partner will delight in the silky softness of it.[32] The hair in the female armpit, if allowed to grow, is very fine and silky and it holds scents longer than a bare axilla.[33] Interestingly, shaving armpit hair probably began as a sexual turn-on.[34]

Body hair dressing has advantages over activities such as body painting. Pubic and armpit hair can be twirled, combed, braided, trimmed, shaped, shaved and dyed. Body painting must be done shortly before SexAct begins (or it will fade or smear). It shows through most clothing and thus can't be worn at work.[35] You can't really do it in the morning, wear it all day and then reveal it to your partner in the evening. Still, it is as much fun for your partner to paint your body as shave it (and less dangerous).[36] And body painting is more easily reversed: if you are unexpectedly invited to a pool party, you can simply wash off the paint; you can't regrow body hair in a couple of hours.[37] There is certainly ample precedent for body painting. During World War 2, when nylon stockings were difficult to obtain, women painted their legs to look as if they were wearing stockings.[38]

A shaved body part requires maintenance; otherwise, the stubble that results can be a problem. You may find it itchy and your partner will probably find it to be a "turn off."[39] Finally, you will not be able to perform *pattes d'araignèe* (literally "spider's legs") if you shave your body hair. This is a form of "massage" in which the hands very, very lightly skim over the surface of the skin just barely touching the fine hair that covers the body. It is very pleasing, but without body hair nothing happens.

We should point out that goosebumps will form whether you shave your body hair or not. Goosebumps develop when tiny muscles contract in order to raise body hair, in order to trap air so as to keep the skin warm. The muscles won't know there is no hair sticking above the skin's surface, so you will get just as many goosebumps. Actually, you may get more because without body hair the skin's surface temperature may be a bit lower and thus the temperature sensors in the skin will register cold more often. As Caesar said in *Bellum Gallicum,* "*in bello parvis momentis magni casus intercedunt*":[40] a goosebump may not expend much energy, but there are thousands of them on a chilly body and they CAN contribute to weight loss.[41]

Opinions about what constitutes sexy change over the years as do attitudes about the amount of hair and where it should be located.[42] Female eyebrows at one time were plucked and shaped, but now, natural, even thick eyebrows are admired. Thus, shaving the pubic region in and of itself is not sexy, nor is shaving the armpits. It is the exotic or forbidden aspect of allowing hair to grow where it is usually removed and vice versa that is exciting. So shaving your eyebrows is currently considered sexy, but it may not be a few years from now.

From our toes to our nose (*a capite ad calcem*), our bodies are covered with hair. Neither shaving body hair nor letting it grow affects energy expenditure.[43] The hair will grow (and use energy doing so) whether you shave or not, assuming you are healthy; hair growth can be retarded by some illnesses and medications. Thus, it should be seen as a technique for enhancing and revitalizing sexual activity. Shaving your partner's initials into your pubic hair (for example) is no weirder than shaving the name of your favorite basketball team onto the back of your head, and young men are doing this and even stranger things everyday. Whether you shave or not makes no difference to your weight loss or maintenance.[44] But it can enhance your sex life.

Not For You, Not For Me, But For Us[45]

Do the best that you can with what you have, whether you are rich or poor, working class or professional, urban or rural. For example, if you are wealthy, you can wear your Laura Ashley hair band, pearls and Rolex. This will add some weight when you are SexExing and thus you will do more work and expend more calories—not many, to be sure, but more than without the hair band, watch and pearls. Of course, a fur coat (a fur jacket is preferable because it leaves you bare from the waist down) weighs more than a string of pearls and will cause you to expend even more calories.

If you are on a limited budget, you can also use what you have. Simply wearing two or more pairs of panty hose during SexEx will add weight and cause your body to work to keep you cool. Of course, they will have to be removed for intercourse, but this can become part of foreplay (let your partner do it). Alternatively, you can simply cut a hole in the crotch (be sure they have a cotton panel or they will unravel and rip). If you can afford it, you can purchase split-crotch panties and panty hose from a number of mail-order vendors.

We are attracted to a person for many reasons—intelligence, personality, and wealth. However, appearance is the major element of sexual attraction.[46] So a concern with appearance and dressing is very important to successful Swell-Wimp, especially if you have a long-time partner.[47] Familiarity breeds contempt or at least boredom and indifference: one must watch out for the Coolidge Effect.[48] You must make yourself appealing to your partner just as you want him or her to be appealing to you.

Chapter 8

Strength and Muscle Control

There are several techniques that can be used during SexEx to increase caloric expenditure. However, before discussing them, we must describe some exercises for increasing strength and muscle control.

First, let us say again that you should not use drugs, such as anabolic steroids, to increase muscle mass and strength. You don't necessarily want that kind of strength; being able to bench press 350 pounds won't help you lose weight or necessarily increase the pleasures of SexAct. Further, steroids are dangerous: they can cause atrophy of the testicles of males; increased body hair growth and lowering of the voice of females; and severe acne on the back and decreased sexual drive in both sexes. Further, they are expensive[1] and illegal.[2]

Some activities (for example, weight lifting) although they require a knowledge of technique, primarily require strength. Other activities require, not strength, but muscle control. A gymnast, for example, although in good physical condition and quite strong, is successful because he or she can control with exquisite precision many of the muscle groups of the body, and thus, he or she is able to balance, roll, spin, turn, revolve, and so on.[3] Sexual activity requires some strength. Both partners must be able to thrust adequately and support their weight on their feet/arms, knees, and elbows. Males also need to support the weight of the female when some of the standing sexual positions are used. Generally though, sexual activity requires control.[4] Strong muscles alone result only in ineffective gross movements.

The Importance of the Back

Strength exercises for the back (especially the lower back) and the pelvic muscles should be done. During sexual climax different things happen in males and females, but in both the back and pelvic muscles play an important role. The male's pelvic muscles thrust the penis deeper into the vagina and the back involuntarily arches driving the entire body forward. The female's back also arches and her pelvis lunges during orgasm.

The back is covered with a complex of muscles running from the neck to the buttocks. In the neck region, there are the Sternocleidomastoid, Sternohyoid, Splenius capitis and Levator scapulae muscles. Around the shoulder blades and upper back, we find the Trapezius, Infraspinatus, Bollix mallanga, Supraspinatus, and Teres major muscles. In the rib region, there are the Latissimus dorsi, Rhomboideus, and Serratus posterior muscles. In the lower back and buttocks region, are located the Abdominal oblique, Gluteus medius, Gluteus maximus, Gluteus minimus, Sirenomelus fickens, Gemellus superior, Foutre bezoar, Obturator internus muscles and the Lumbodorsal fascia. All of these must work efficiently and together on both sides of the body or you may incur a strain, pull, or tear.

One of the most common ailments today is "a back problem"; everybody has, or knows someone who has, one. Atual Gawande claims that "Chronic back pain is now second only to the common cold as a cause of lost work time and it accounts for forty per cent of workers'-compensation payments."[5] A "back problem" can be tremendously painful and almost impossible to cure. Frequently you don't know what caused it; you just say "I pulled my back," or "I popped something in my back," but you can't really point to the time or cause of the injury. Millions of dollars are lost every year because people miss work and additional millions are spent on pills, creams, heating pads, braces, surgery and various other treatments. According to Richard A. Deyo "medicine has at best a limited understanding of the condition. In fact, medicine's reliance on outdated ideas may actually contribute to the problem." And "there are no differences in functional recovery times among patients who saw chiropractors, family doctors or orthopedic surgeons." That is, neither bed rest nor surgery nor manual manipulation nor traction seems to make a difference in most cases.[6] So if "back problems" cannot be treated, they should be prevented.

Many back injuries occur during SexAct.[7] You have almost no conscious control of the back and pelvic muscles during climax, yet they flex strenuously. Pain and stiffness may not develop until 24 to 48 hours after the injury occurs. Thus, you don't associate the pain with SexAct. You assume that you must have lifted something incorrectly, using your back instead of your legs, but that's not usually the cause.

Deyo points out that the "American economy is increasingly post-industrial, with less heavy labor, more automation and more robotics, and medicine has consistently improved diagnostic imaging of the spine and developed new forms of surgical and non-surgical therapy. But work disability caused by back pain has steadily risen."[8] One hundred years ago when a greater proportion of the population earned its living doing physical labor, there were far fewer back problems. Were they more intelligent? That is, did more of them know how to lift with their legs instead of their backs? No, we are as smart as they. But their backs were in better shape: they used their backs more so the muscles were stronger and thus they injured themselves less frequently during SexAct.[9] If you are going to engage in SexActs that result in climax, you should have a strong back[10] and "there is growing evidence for exercise as an important part of the prevention and treatment of back problems."[11]

How do you strengthen your back? As was pointed out earlier, exercises to strengthen the shoulders (pushups) and neck (neck arches) are good. Back arches, which build up all of the back muscles somewhat, are very good. To do them, lie on the floor belly down and place your arms at your sides. Then lift your head and legs off the floor simultaneously (do not use your hands). If you can't raise both head and legs at the same time, lift them alternately. If you can raise them simultaneously, rock back and forth on your belly (back arches now become belly rolls). You should start back arches slowly since you do not want to cause a problem while trying to prevent one. Start with two or three and work up to fifty or seventy-five.

Pelvic thrusts are good for the lower-back and pelvic muscles. Stand upright, feet apart about shoulder width, arms akimbo. While holding your upper body still and straight, pivot your pelvis forward as though you were thrusting during intercourse. Your knees will bend slightly and your buttocks will tighten. At first this may seem awkward and you will not get a good thrust (more like a rocking forward), but with practice you will look like the best of the "dirty dancers." There is no need to start slowly: begin with about fifty and progress quickly to two hundred.

When you have strengthened the back somewhat, you are ready for another exercise which strengthens the legs, buttocks, back and shoulders simultaneously. You need a partner to do this. Lie face down across a bed (perpendicular to the direction in which you sleep). Slide forward until your body from the waist up is hanging off the bed. Have your partner press your legs down on the bed. Now lift your body from a hanging position until the top half is level with the bottom half. This is a very good exercise since you are lifting about half of your body weight with your back, buttock and leg muscles, but you should not try it until your back has already been strengthened. Any flat object that is raised a couple of feet off the floor or ground can be used: a table, couch, desk, freezer chest, workbench, boat dock, car hood, porch, hay wagon, or steam table. Thus, you can do it almost anywhere (although you need someone or something to hold your legs down).[12]

This exercise can be combined with intercourse *a tergo*[13] and it is both effective and pleasurable if both partners synchronize their movements. Since you are close to the edge, be careful not to tumble off.

Gochros points out that "sexual activity itself is an excellent form of exercise therapy for the back, stomach and pelvic muscles and if undertaken in a regular and reasonably vigorous manner can help reduce back pain" (33). Thus, if you have a bad back, doing the exercises we have recommended will strengthen your back, making you fitter for SexEx. SexEx, which, in turn, will further strengthen your back, enabling you to do even more exercises and SexEx. Isn't it wonderful the way feedback loops work?

The Breasts

There are no muscles in the breasts which are actually enlarged, specialized diaphoretic glands. The milk is a specialized form of sweat, enriched with proteins from the mother's blood.[14] Thus, there are no exercises to strengthen the breast muscles (because they do not exist).[15] Neither are there exercises to increase the size of the breasts. During puberty, a girl's breasts blossom and grow to their adult size.[16] They usually increase in size during pregnancy as they prepare for nursing the newborn baby. As long as the baby is nursed, the breasts maintain their size (or even grow larger). After the child is weaned, the breasts shrink, but usually not to their pre-pregnancy size. There are no exercises that make the breasts larger.[17] Any exercise that develops the underlying muscles (Pectoralis major and minor) will raise the breasts higher off the chest wall, but the breasts themselves do not get bigger. There is far too much concern with breasts in American society;[18] although they are sensitive to fondling and sucking, they are not the primary sex organ.[19] So, be satisfied with what you have (or your partner has) and devote your exercise time to developing those things that you can (and should) do something about.[20]

Vagina

During arousal, the spongy tissues around the labia minora and majora swell and grow turgid.[21] The walls of the vagina ooze a slippery substance; this occurs because vasocongestion[22] the vaginal lining in a process called transudation.[23] Engorgement of the vulva increases the effective length of the vaginal canal[24] and thus the size of the penis it can accommodate; it also brings the clitoris and labia minora, sexually sensitive structures, into closer contact with the penis. The clitoris[25] becomes erect and sticks out from its foreskin.

Orgasm is marked by simultaneous rhythmic muscular contractions of the uterus, the outer third of the vagina and the anal sphincter. Mild orgasm may have three to five contractions and intense orgasm may have ten to fifteen. After orgasm, the pelvic veins empty rapidly.

Although a woman cannot regulate blood flow into the various structures, she can control her vaginal muscles to some extent and the more she can do this (and the fitter these muscles are), the more she can enhance her and her partner's pleasure.

Several "vaginal" muscles are important for SexEx. The bulbocavernosus or vaginal sphincter muscle is split into halves, one on each side of the vaginal opening. As it contracts, the vagina is almost squeezed shut. The urethral sphincter, whose major purpose is to shut off urine flow, also compresses the vagina just inside the vaginal opening. When the levator ani group, which extends from the anal to the pubic area and surrounds the deeper part of the vagina, is constricted, the walls of the vagina are brought together and, during intercourse, the penis is squeezed along its entire length. If the man keeps his penis motionless within the vagina, the woman can massage its entire length by contracting these muscles. In centuries past, trained Indian women were able to bring a man to climax using this technique.[26]

When a woman contracts the external sphincter muscles (as if refraining from urinating), the sensitive nerve endings at the vaginal opening are stimulated, the clitoris is expanded and thus the woman's pleasure is increased.

Females can strengthen their vaginal muscles by using the same Kegel exercises[27] that are used to warm them up: repeatedly tighten and release the muscles that control micturition and defecation.[28] You can feel a kind of internal lifting as you tighten. The contractions should be held only for a few seconds and be repeated daily for at least one hundred contractions to be effective. You can do Kegels almost anywhere and anytime; no one in the check-out line will know you are exercising. When you have strengthened the muscles and learned to control them consciously, you will be able to "grab" the penis inside you and even "massage" it. Doing this, of course, pleases the male, but it gives you even more pleasure: contracting the muscles to grab the penis brings the vaginal walls into contact with the penis; as it moves forward and backward, it strokes the vagina.[29]

Clitoris

It has been proved that all female orgasms are the result of clitoral stimulation (direct or indirect). There is really no such thing as a distinct vaginal (Freudian) orgasm, although the sensations during orgasm resulting from masturbation can be different from those resulting from intercourse.

The clitoris has at least the same number of nerve cells as, and is as responsive to stimulation as, the much larger penis. Rubbing it and tugging the labia minora (which applies a tug to the clitoris) arouses it. The male erection takes place outside the body and is more visible than the female's, but the total size of female engorgement is no smaller than that of an erect penis. If a woman loses her clitoris due to surgery or initiation mutilation (as in Somalia), she can still achieve orgasm since many of the clitoral nerves remain.

It is a myth that woman are slower to respond than men. When women masturbate, they climax as quickly as men, but during intercourse there is not as much stimulation to the clitoris.[30] So in old-fashioned SexAct, it seemed that the woman was slow to climax (if she did at all). Some cultures don't even acknowledge that women can enjoy SexAct let alone achieve orgasm.[31] During intercourse, orgasm usually results from indirect stimulation of the clitoris by the male genitalia and from conscious effort by the woman to achieve stimulation of the clitoral area. The woman-on-top position is good for this, although it doesn't guarantee an orgasm.[32]

As far as we can determine, women have no more control of the movement of "the little man in the boat" than men do of their penises. Because of its small size, no exercises are recommended, although development of the bulbocavernosus and levator ani muscles are useful (see below).

The Penis

Many people are surprised to learn that the average penis is only about six inches long with the normal range running from four and one-half inches to eight inches.[33] In Alabama, belief in the Dew Willie is still current—a penis long enough to be wetted by the dew during urination outside in the morning and evening. However, since it is the tip of the penis that requires stimulation for orgasm to occur, even a very short penis is stimulated sufficiently during intercourse. The notion that a bigger penis is better is contrary to the mechanics of male and female pleasure; a longer penis does not mean more pleasure for either. There are no methods for permanently increasing its length or circumference and there is no need to.[34]

The penis becomes erect when cavities within it fill with blood—a hydraulic action.[35] Therefore, it is important that the cardiovascular system be in good shape for a fast, hard, long-lasting erection. Animals reach orgasm quickly but men are not animals[36] and premature ejaculation is not normal or desirable. Most males can continue intercourse for five or ten minutes during which time they deliver fifty to one hundred thrusts.[37]

Unfortunately, human males can move the penis only a small distance toward the abdomen. It can be pleasurable for the male to enter the woman, but refrain from thrusting, substituting for a while, only the upward movement of the penis. Since this activity expends energy, it can be used to increase weight loss. However, if carried on too long it may result in fatigue and impatience (both partners), so employ it as one of several pre-orgasmic activities.

Constricting the levator ani group thrusts the penis forward and temporarily increases its length. The action of trying to hold back a bowel movement strengthens this group. Contracting the bulbocavernosus muscle compresses the erectile tissues of the penis and causes an increase in diameter. Although, the contraction can be held for only a few seconds, the woman can feel the increase in size within her. Males should also do Kegel exercises.

Although the penis can't be made permanently larger, the muscles that control it can be made stronger. A simple exercise is to place weights on the head of the erect penis and then lift the penis upward by flexing the same muscles that are used to stop urination. You can use pennies (or other coins), a wrist watch or something similar. The exercise works best if the weight is placed on the head of the penis rather than on the shaft. Try to lift increasingly heavier weights and try for speed (make it bob up and down quickly). There is no need to buy or construct special weights; in fact, a glazed doughnut works exceptionally well, since its stickiness helps it to stay on the penis.[38] When the exercise period is over, a transition to foreplay is made when your partner removes the doughnut by eating it.[39]

Testicles

The testicles produce sperm and the male hormone testosterone; without testicles and thus without testosterone, sexual events are inhibited. If they are lost before puberty, a sexually undeveloped male (eunuch) results. If the testicles are lost or cease to function after puberty, ejaculation and intercourse are still possible, since the penis is still sensitive to stimulation, the seminal vesicles still produce fluid and the two adrenal glands produce some testosterone.

When climax occurs, the urethra is sealed off and secretions from the prostate gland, seminal vesicles and testicles mix. A man ejaculates 1/4 ounce of seminal fluid in about six spurts.[40] The prostate gland adds a secretion which increases the activity of the sperm.[41] The Cowper's glands produce the pre-ejaculatory drops of fluid (each containing about 50,000 sperm) that seep from the penis during erection. Thus, even if ejaculation doesn't occur inside the female, pregnancy can result because the pre-ejaculatory fluid on the head of the penis carries sperm into the vagina. So use birth control.

Sperm production requires a temperature a few degrees below the normal body temperature of 98.6, so the testicles hang outside of the body where they can be cooled. When it is cold, the skin shrinks and draws the testicles closer to the body where they are warmed.[42] Thousands of years ago men had strong muscles in the skin of the scrotum that could pull the testicles up into the abdomen where they were protected from injury.[43] Today, we are able to voluntarily lift them only slightly (as when a physician says "Cough"); otherwise, they move closer or farther from the body involuntarily. During climax they are drawn up toward the body, but there is no reason to try to develop this ability. It will not result in increased pleasure or weight loss.

Vasocongestion, due to sexual arousal, causes the testicles to swell and become 50% to 100% larger than in the unstimulated state. There are no known methods of increasing the size of the testicles,[45] but this is not a problem since size is not related to potency either in terms of sexual performance or sperm production and it has no bearing upon the degree of pleasure during SexAct or weight loss during Swell-Wimp.

The Tongue

One of the most important muscles associated with sexual activity is the tongue; it comes into play so very often—during fellatio, cunnilingus, kissing, and licking.[46] Although most are naturally strong, every tongue can be strengthened. Further, few people are able to fully control their tongues.[47] We recommend the following exercises. The male should lie on his back with, at least, a semierect penis. His partner positions herself face down over the penis straddling his chest (facing his feet) and places the top side of her tongue on the head of the penis. She then forces the penis toward the man's feet and to the right and left.

Then she straddles his legs (facing his head) and repeats the exercises with the underside of her tongue. This is more difficult because the tongue is strongest when moving outward and/or upward. However, the underside of the tongue is smoother and can give more pleasure, so both exercises should be done.[48]

This exercise also benefits the male (aside from the pleasure he derives from it). He should attempt to resist the pressure of his partner's tongue—easily done when she is pressing downward—by tightening the muscles associated with micturition and defecation. However, resisting the lateral movements is very difficult and only with practice can he achieve any control and strength here. But the effort is worth it; being able to move the penis, not only upward but also sideways in his partner's vagina will enhance the pleasure of both immensely.

A man's tongue can be strengthened by attempting to separate the labia majora and penetrate the vagina while the woman resists. He should try this facing toward her head and then facing her feet (using the underside of his tongue). The woman must carefully regulate the degree to which she resists, since it is easy for her to prevent any penetration by the tongue and he might smother if she catches and holds his nose.[44]

These exercises expend considerable calories (although it would not seem so); they build strength and they develop control.[49]

The Nose

The male nose can be an instrument of sexual pleasure if controlled properly.[50] Generally, it is used with the tongue during cunnilingus to stimulate the clitoris.[51] He must control his excitement and remember that a nose is composed of bone and cartilage; many men's naric appendages stick out farther than their tongues. He can easily hurt his partner if his nose too forcefully thrusts against sensitive tissues. Further, he must be careful not to introduce mucous excretions (snot) into the vulva or vagina, especially if he has a cold or other communicable disease.

During arousal, the soft parts of the nose, the alea, become swollen and so the nostrils expand.[52] Except for flaring the nostrils, humans have little control of the movements of the nose. Narial exercises to strengthen the muscles that flare the nostrils are, as far as we know, useless.[53]

The Cardiovascular System

The cardiovascular system plays an important role in good sexual performance. The penis contains cavities which when filled with blood result in an erection. A weak cardiovascular system can result in a weak, slow or brief erection.[54] There have been cases in which men with unusually large penises have passed out whenever they got an erection because their hearts were unable to maintain adequate blood pressure. None of the men are reported to have sustained serious injury from the falls. Occasionally, women with weak hearts become light-headed and even faint when sexually aroused. Therefore, any exercise that improves the cardiovascular system can be beneficial to SexEx.

The best way to improve the cardiovascular system is to do aerobic exercises which raise the pulse and respiration rates substantially above normal for more than a brief period. Additionally, twenty minutes of aerobic exercise burns three hundred calories. For most people, SexAct is not aerobic. The pulse rate is elevated to 160 beats per minute or more and blood pressure can double, but only during climax. Thus, SexAct is not truly aerobic. But SexEx can be.[55] There is no reason that you cannot do your strengthening and warm-up exercises strenuously enough to make them aerobic.

Conclusion

All of exercises discussed in this chapter are excellent. They can be done naked or with additional clothing (see Chapter 7) in order to burn extra calories. Better control will result in more pleasure for you and your partner, especially if you synchronize your muscle contractions for mutual stimulation. However, as Seneca said, *nemo liber est qui corpori servit.*[56] You don't want to become muscle bound. This occurs when muscle-building activity results in some muscles interfering with the movement of other muscles. It is a well-known fact that many body builders cannot swim because they do not have adequate freedom of movement of the arms and shoulders. Certainly, you do not want to become unnaturally overdeveloped—for example, a tongue so large and strong that your speech is affected. Swell-Wimp should be easy, NATURAL, and fun. Further, too much exercise can result in excessive loss of body fat (some body fat is normal) and in women this can result in cessation of menstruation (which may or may not be desirable). Thus, as we have said before, be moderate.[57] Exercise to lose weight and to develop muscles that will enhance the pleasure of SexAct, but don't overdo.

Chapter 9

Oops!

Sometimes sexual activity can result in weight gain![1] In addition to being pleasurable, intercourse is a procreative activity; that's how babies are made.[2] It is beyond the scope of this book to fully explain the procreative process. Basically, sperm from the male are injected into the female where they search out the female egg.[3] The sperm unites with (fertilizes) the egg and then the egg travels to the uterus where for nine[4] months it grows to become a baby. If you are engaging in intercourse for pleasure, you should, as Dr. Ruth frequently reminds us, "use protection." That is, use some method or device to prevent conception and thus pregnancy.[5] Read the following statistics carefully, especially if you are a teenager. In 1982, Masters, Johnson and Kolodny reported that there were thirty thousand pregnancies each year among girls under the age of fifteen. Four-hundred thousand teenagers have abortions each year (one-third of all abortions). Sixty percent of teenage females who have a child before seventeen will be pregnant again before nineteen. The United States teenage birth rate is the highest in the western hemisphere.[6] These statistics reflect a lot of ignorance about sex and conception and a lot of messed-up lives (mothers and babies).[7] And they are about two decades old; things are worse today. There is no need to become pregnant if you don't want to and yes it is more complicated than just saying no. We won't attempt to give a comprehensive discussion of birth-control methods—just a brief overview. There are numerous places where you can obtain accurate and reliable information. Some methods of birth control may be inconvenient but the possibility of cyesis can cast a shadow over the enjoyment of SexAct. And pregnancy can cast a permanent shadow over your entire life. If you are sexually active, USE BIRTH CONTROL.[8]

Abstinence This method runs directly counter to the thesis of this book. However, it is the most effective method for preventing pregnancy and for avoiding sexually-transmitted diseases. Give it some thought and discuss it with your partner before dismissing it.[9]

Rhythm This "natural" method relies on the fact that a woman is more likely to become pregnant at certain times during her monthly cycle. It requires daily tracking of the female's temperature and engaging in SexAct only on specific days. The method doesn't really work very well, but it is the only method of birth control approved by the Catholic Church.[10]

Douching This method requires using an apparatus to wash out the vagina with a solution immediately after intercourse. David Ruben claims that Coca-Cola works well because the carbonic acid kills sperm, the sugar explodes the sperm cells and the carbonation forces the stuff into the tiny crevices of the vaginal lining.[11] You can also purchase prepared douches at a pharmacy. However, by the time douching is started, very many sperm are already in the uterus. Further, having to carry douching equipment around with you kills spontaneity and jumping up to douche immediately after intercourse prohibits any period of languorous intimacy or re-arousal. Douching is better than nothing, but not by much.

Diaphragm A diaphragm is a cap that is inserted at the end of the cervix to prevent sperm from traveling further. It is about 90% effective, and can be inserted long before intercourse. But you do have to remember to carry it with you or insert it every morning and it can sometimes fall out or have pinholes in it.

IUD: Intra-uterine device This is a device that is placed in the uterus and left there. It is about 90% effective and you don't have to put it in just before sex. But it may cause some bleeding, discomfort, and cramping. Some manufacturers' IUDs have caused even worse problems and their use has resulted in permanent damage to the users.

IPD: Intra-penal device There is no such thing, yet. Judy Small's "The IPD Song" is fiction.

Condom Called "perseverativo" in Spain, "capote" in France and "Weinersheathen" in Germany, they are about 85% effective. They afford some protection against sexually-transmitted disease, and are available almost everywhere at any time (there are vending machines in many rest rooms). But condoms can have microscopic holes in them and they are destroyed by petroleum jelly (use water-soluble jelly). They have four drawbacks: a small percentage of men are allergic to the materials from which condoms are made;[12] they have to be put on just prior to intercourse; they lessen male sensitivity (so men don't like them); they are the only birth-control device used by men. However, there is no reason why a woman can't carry condoms with her and INSIST that the male use them.

Vaginal suppository The first recorded prescriptions for limiting fertility (in the Kahun Medical Papyrus, an Egyptian document circa 1850 BC), are for vaginal suppositories.[13] Suppositories contain chemicals that prevent conception and must be placed in the vagina before intercourse. You must carry them with you and sometimes they don't melt sufficiently, and even if they do, many sperm don't come into contact with the spermicide.

Vaginal foam Like suppositories, foams chemically prevent conception. You must carry the container of foam with you and spray it into the vagina just prior to intercourse.

Anal intercourse Mme de Réan-Fichini points out that this is a sure-fire method of avoiding conception,[14] but that is all. It can damage the lower intestinal tract and offers little chance of orgasm for the woman. And because the rectal mucosa bleed easily, blood and semen often mix—an excellent way to transmit diseases, including AIDS.[15]

Birth-control pill If taken correctly oral contraceptives are about 98% effective. They work by altering the female's reproductive chemistry. Oral contraceptives, which must be taken daily, have been on the market for a long time and there are studies showing that they do and do not cause long-term problems. The consensus is that they are safe, but you should have regular checkups.[16] Another form of birth-control that works as oral contraceptives do by altering the reproductive chemistry requires the insertion of several capsules beneath the skin. It is effective for months at a time, thus eliminating one of the biggest problems with the pill—the need to remember to take them every day. These implants should be as safe and effective as the birth-control pill, but they have been available for only a short time so their long-term safety is unknown.

Oral contraceptives have proven to be safe and effective over three decades of use. Given this, why are they so expensive? They now cost about $30.00 per pack ($1.00 per day).[17] The price of a drug is determined in part by the need to recoup development costs (sometimes many millions of dollars), but surely that happened a decade or two ago. Built into the price is some amount that is set aside for potential legal costs, but after three decades the legal-costs escrow accounts must be bulging. Further, they are manufactured by the billions (economy of scale) and there is no shortage of manufacturing capacity (the "law" of supply and demand), so over the years the price should have gone down, but it has actually gone up. The economy is booming and inflation is virtually nil, yet I've just been informed that again my prescription will cost more next month. Are women being forced to subsidize the development of other drugs—such as Viagra? Still, $30.00 per month isn't much compared to the grief and expense of an unwanted pregnancy.[18]

Not every couple can use every birth-control method.[19] There are other methods that we haven't discussed and continuing research may provide better birth-control options. There may be physical, psychological or religious reasons that prevent a man or woman from using one method or another. Some require a prescription, some are more effective and some are more expensive. You should talk to your sexual partner about which method to use and to a birth-control counselor or physician for more information about the risks and benefits of any method before you try it.

Dual Responsibility

Both men and women are responsible for birth control. A vasectomy is a surgical procedure in which a section of the vas deferens (the duct that carries sperm from the testicles to the ejaculatory duct) is excised in order to produce permanent sterilization in a man.[20] A vasectomy does not require the removal of the testicles. It is a relatively inexpensive and simple procedure that can be done in a physician's office under local anesthetic and there is almost no pain (only a little soreness for a couple of days). A man who has had a vasectomy is not less virile nor is his sex drive diminished.[21] Tubal ligation is a procedure by which the Fallopian tubes are cut and tied so that eggs can't travel to the uterus; the woman is made permanently sterile.[22] A woman is no less feminine nor is her sex drive diminished after tubal ligation. However, it is a more expensive and serious medical procedure than vasectomy with a greater risk of complications.

If, for whatever reason, you have decided that you do not want children (or more children), you should seriously consider permanent sterilization. SexAct can be more spontaneous and enjoyable when you do not have the ever-present fear of becoming pregnant or causing pregnancy. You no longer have to carry birth-control devices with you. Also, the female does not have the additional worries that result from long-term use of some birth control methods. However, even though you have been permanently sterilized, if you have not settled into a single-partner relationship, you should still use condoms (male or female), since they are the only proven method of reducing your chances of contracting AIDS or a venereal disease.

We don't advocate coitus interruptus, posterior urethral compression or Karezza as methods of avoiding conception during intercourse. Basically, Karezza is a technique whereby intercourse continues for a long time without ejaculation. It has been used to treat men who ejaculate as soon as (or soon after) the penis enters the vagina. It was used by the Oneida community as a method of providing sexual pleasure while avoiding pregnancies. Something similar was used by the Taoists for preserving the spiritual energy they believed resided in semen.[23] Coitus interruptus involves removing the penis from the vagina prior to ejaculation.

As we have pointed out before, prior to ejaculation a drop or two of secretion containing about 50,000 sperm leaves the penis. Thus, any birth-control method that allows for the insertion of the erect penis into the vagina brings with it the chance of pregnancy even though the penis is removed before ejaculation.

Posterior urethral compression requires squeezing the penis at its base just at the moment of ejaculation, thus forcing the semen back into the prostate gland and seminal vesicles. It is painful and damaging and like *coitus interruptus* and Karezza it does not prevent sperm from entering the vagina before ejaculation.[24]

Shere Hite reports that several studies have shown there is a better chance of getting pregnant if the woman does not have an orgasm.[25] This makes no sense as a birth-control method: the possibility of pregnancy is lessened only slightly and there are few occasions when a woman would willingly engage in SexAct without orgasm. Also, keep in mind that, although conception is less likely while a woman is lactating, it is not impossible or uncommon, so don't think you can't get pregnant just because you are currently nursing a baby.

A Flower in Your Apron

It is interesting to note that we don't have many terms for pregnancy. There are, of course, "expecting" (we don't ask "What?"), "preggers" and the slightly old-fashioned "with child" and "in a family way." And there are the cruder euphemisms, such as "knocked up,"[26] "caught," "bun in the oven," and "up the stump." This says something about us (English-speaking people) and what we value. Our literary language has thousands of figures of speech (similes, metaphors, and so on) for war, bravery, beauty, and death, but almost none for conception, pregnancy or birth. For some reason pregnancy has been an unspeakable condition.[27]

We propose a new metaphor—"a flower in [her, my, your] apron." For example, "My wife has a flower in her apron" or "Jane! Do you have a flower in your apron?" This metaphor is derived from D. H. Lawrence's short story "Odour of Chrysanthemums." In the story the phrase is spoken to a mother by her young daughter who does not yet know her mother is pregnant. "Flower" and "flowering" connote beautiful, fragile, growing things[28] and "apron" carries with it the associations of motherhood, nurturing, work and protection.[29]

Conclusion

There is a TV commercial for automotive oil filters that makes its point when a mechanic says, "You can pay me now or pay me later." The cost of regularly changing your oil and filter is much less than paying a mechanic to rebuild your car's engine. Birth control is like this. It is cheap when compared to the cost of bearing and raising a child. Also, if you don't really want children (because of age, financial situation or whatever), pregnancy can have a tremendous psychological cost. And the psychological costs to an unwanted child are incalculable.

If you find that you have a flower in your apron, see a physician immediately. Start or continue pre-natal care. You should be able to continue Swell-Wimp until the sixth month of your pregnancy, but discuss the subject with your physician. Of course, follow her or his advice about diet, exercise, and medications. If you are a drug user—alcohol, nicotine, tranquilizers, marijuana, cocaine, heroine, barbiturates, amphetamines, or anything else—for the health of your baby, stop "using" immediately.

We believe that sex may be engaged in for pleasure only, but the participants should be aware of the possibility that conception can occur. Pregnancy is not something that should happen by accident.[30] Yes, we know that some people argue that whether you conceive or not is up to God or Allah or whom/whatever and that it is wrong to try to thwart his/her/its plan. Well, it may be God's plan to have you run over by a garbage truck, but you still look both ways before crossing the street. There are so many people on this earth (especially in China and India), the birth rate is so high (in Mexico and several other developing nations), and we are depleting the planet's resources (in the Western industrialized nations and especially in the United States) and destroying the environment so quickly (everywhere) that it is irresponsible not to use birth control measures unless you WANT to conceive and (this is important) you are in a position (financial, social, and psychological) to raise the child that results (not leave it to God, society or mom and dad). We take a pro-choice position regarding abortion,[31] but we do not consider (and you should not either) abortion to be a birth-control method. It is an extreme measure to be used only when absolutely necessary. Thus, whenever you engage in SexAct, you should be prepared for the possibility of conception (and years of caring for a child). With a few precautions Swell-Wimp can be easy, natural and fun.

Chapter 10
Techniques

Finally, we come to the techniques that can be used to increase calorie expenditure and thus enhance weight loss. There are important differences between men and women regarding strength, speed, and stamina. Men, in general, are stronger and have greater burst speed than women. Although we usually associate men with marathon running, around-the-world sailing, mountain climbing and making war, women actually have greater physical stamina.[1] Also, their fine muscle control is better, and they live longer. Men are stronger in the upper body; women are stronger in the thighs and pelvic region. Of course, any individual may deviate from the average: a woman may be stronger than a man who may have greater muscle control than a woman. Each of the following exercises is designed to be done by men and women, with necessary changes pointed out for each sex. Still, the lack of strength by women and the lack of endurance by men may give the other sex an advantage (especially obvious if you are doing the exercises together). You should not let this lead to frustration. SexEx is not Swell-Wimp if it is not easy, natural and FUN. The exercises are meant to be a part of Swell-Wimp, not challenges in and of themselves.

Sit-Ups

One of our favorite exercises is sexual sit-ups. Females do them in the missionary position: man on top, face-to-face with both partners stretched to full length (no legs on shoulders or top of torso hanging off the bed).[2] After entering her, the man sits up as far as he can without causing himself or his partner pain, placing his legs in a comfortable position. Then the woman does sit-ups, placing her arms and hands alongside her body (least difficult), behind her head or across her chest (most difficult).[3]

Male sexual sit-ups begin in the reverse missionary position (man on the bottom). The woman slips the penis into her vagina and she raises herself until she is sitting astraddle the man, leaning forward a little so as not to cause herself or her partner discomfort (her legs will be folded alongside the man's hips). He then performs sit-ups, perhaps kissing one of her breasts each time. The man's hands and arms can be placed behind his head, along side his body or across his chest.

During sexual sit-ups, the top partners may have to lean backward somewhat and even place their hands on the other's shins in order to achieve balance. The person sitting up can wear wrist weights or hold something in his or her arms (a pillow, book, puppy or toaster, for example) to make the sit-ups even more difficult and thus use even more calories.

Sexual sit-ups are very stimulating (both partners) and, like regular sit-ups, strengthen the stomach muscles and expend a lot of calories. However, be sure to roll or curl your upper body forward and upward as you rise. It should not be held rigid; this can cause the stomach muscles to tear. The one doing the sit-ups must be careful so as not to konk[4] the partner's head or chest.

There is a static (isometric) variation of the sexual sit-up that expends additional calories, but is more difficult and has a greater risk of injury. The partner on the bottom lies with his or her upper body (down to about the waist) off the edge of the bed.[5] He or she then holds his or her body horizontal as they continue SexAct.[6] Placing the hands behind the head makes this exercise even more difficult. This technique should be tried only after the stomach muscles have been strengthened, since failure to keep yourself horizontal will cause you to flop over the edge of the bed which can result in head injury, dizziness, blackout, and back injury. Also, you should not try to do sit-ups by allowing yourself to drape down over the edge of the bed and then raise yourself to the horizontal position unless your stomach and back muscles are very strong, since this can easily result in a muscle tear. This kind of sit-up burns a lot of calories; even the upper partner must work hard to remain upright or both will tumble off the bed. Because of the risk of injury, some of the subjects of our study found this technique very stimulating; they felt they were performing "on the edge."

Another variation of the sexual sit-up is the neck lift. Place yourself (as the lower partner) so that your shoulders are just at the edge of the bed with your head hanging over. Then raise your head all the way. This is very good for the neck muscles and there is little risk of injury unless you allow your head to rapidly flop backward or raise your head too quickly and konk your partner.

Leg Lifts

Sexual leg lifts are very good for the stomach and leg muscles. Male leg lifts are done in the reverse missionary position.[7] The woman leans over the man and supports herself on her hands, knees and toes (which are placed outside the man's hips). The man brings his legs together (side-by-side and straight), slowly raises them six to twelve inches and then lowers them.

Female leg lifts are identical except that the woman is on the bottom. They are a bit more difficult, since her closed legs will squeeze the man's penis tightly, and when she lifts them, they will press against his scrotum. There is little risk of injury or pain, unless the leg lifts are performed too rapidly. Many people find this exercise very pleasurable.

The first few times you do leg lifts, do them on the floor or some other hard (but padded) surface, since the softness of the bed prevents good back support which makes the exercise more difficult and increases the risk of injury.

Since, during leg lifts, the lower partner does not sit up, the upper partner should lean forward over the lower and support some of his or her weight on his or her arms and thus place less backward pressure on the penis.

It is also possible for the lower partner to do leg lifts and sit-ups simultaneously, but he or she should not alternate from one to the other because this causes a rocking motion which (1) makes the sit-ups and leg lifts easier and (2) can easily increase in speed and amplitude; such oscillations can cause both partners discomfort and can get out of control so that injury occurs. This is a problem especially if the bed springs are soft or if the exercise is done on a water bed.

Another variation of leg lifts (for both women and men) requires the lower partner (the lifter) to spread his or her legs and the upper to close his or her legs. It is actually easier to lift your legs when they are spread than when held together. In this variation, the man's penis is squeezed when he is doing the leg lifts.

Finally, both partners can do leg lifts simultaneously. They lie on their sides and he enters her from the front or rear. Then they both lift their upper legs either simultaneously or alternately. After forty or fifty lifts, they roll over onto their other sides and repeat the exercise with the other leg. This exercises different muscles than when leg lifts are done on your back. Unlike with most sexual exercises, both partners do the same exercise at the same time.

As with sit-ups, leg lifts can be made more difficult by wearing shoes, boots, or ankle weights to increase the amount of energy expended. When doing leg lifts and sit-ups, you must use common sense. If you have heavy legs or are really out of shape, start slowly and work up to more lifts over a period of weeks. If either of you have large thighs, you should avoid any of the positions that might result in excessive squeezing of the penis or scrotum. If your breasts are large (male or female), you may want to avoid the position in which upper half of your body hangs off the bed, because there may be too much weight for your stomach muscles to handle. If your abdomen(s) is/are large, you may have to experiment a bit to find comfortable positions for sexual sit-ups.

Pushups

Sexual pushups differ somewhat from regular pushups. You support your weight on your hands and knees rather than hands and toes and you bend your body at the waist to achieve a rocking motion rather than keeping your body rigid and horizontal. Pushups can be done with the knees together or spread apart.

Sexual pushups are especially good for women who, in general, are weaker than men in the upper body.[8] In the reverse missionary position, the male can support some of the (upper) woman's weight with his hands, thus making the pushups easier and strengthening his upper body at the same time.[9] Pushups develop the pectoral muscles and this causes the breasts to sit higher off the chest wall and appear larger. However, the gain in size is rather small unless the pushups are done with the dedication of a body-builder; therefore, large-breasted woman need not avoid them because they fear their chest measurement will increase.

A woman can also do pushups from most of the rear-entry positions. She does pushups while her partner helps her (if necessary) by pulling upward and backward on her hips. The complimentary exercise for men is quite difficult. After being entered in the missionary position, the woman wraps her arms around the man's neck or shoulders and her legs around his hips. The man then rises to his hands and knees (supporting the woman who is hanging on to him) and does shallow pushups. Both partners expend considerable energy, but most people find this variation too difficult.[10]

A variation on the sexual pushup was performed by the famous Bedouin warrior, Abu Hasan, who had a dwarf armed with a scimitar crouch on his shoulders when he engaged in intercourse in order to prevent his enemies from sneaking up on him. We don't advise that you do the same, but if you have a pet—a cat or ferret, for example—you could place it on your shoulders or neck during sexual pushups to increase the difficulty.

Clasping the Tree

As you see, traditional calisthenics easily integrate with SexEx. Other adaptations are possible. For example, the partners can assume the position in which the woman (facing the man) wraps her legs around his trunk and then he stands.[11] He can then do deep knee-bends and/or walk up and down the stairs.[12] The extra weight of the woman causes the man to expend additional energy, as does the woman who must hold on and remain steady lest she or her partner injure their sexual organs. Thus, we advise that such combinations be attempted only after you have achieved a moderate degree of fitness and only by those who could endure a loss of sexual pleasure or income for a week or two.

Keep in mind that in this chapter we are focusing on techniques that can be used to burn additional calories DURING, not BEFORE, SexAct. Use your imagination; you can invent many other energy-expending techniques.[13] For example, one partner can do sit-ups, leg lifts or pushups while the other performs cunnilingus or fellatio.

As we have said, there is no need to purchase exercise equipment for Swell-Wimp, but SexEx can be combined with a workout—at home or done at a private[14] health club. We do advise EXTREME caution in combining SexAct with workouts using Nautilus (and similar) equipment. The gleaming chrome, digital displays, and so on can add a certain high-tech stimulus to SexAct and the sound of leather and the motion of suspended weights can add to the sensuality of the experience, but injury is a very real possibility. However, the element of danger can also be stimulating.

Dancing

Dancing is good exercise and fun, and can be done rapidly or slowly. Currently, aerobic dancing is a very popular form of exercise, usually done with several to many people standing in rows facing an instructor. The same kind of bouncy dancing, done dressed or naked, can be integrated into Swell-Wimp. Jitterbugging, square dancing, and even waltzing (at high speed) require considerable energy expenditure.

Many people find contact dancing arousing.[15] And taking off some or all of your clothes while dancing is certainly erotic. Dancing can be used for warming up, as a part of foreplay, and for strength and fitness exercises.[16]

It can also be integrated with coitus. For example, after assuming the Clasping-the-Tree position, the male can dance around the room. Depending upon his strength and agility, he can just shuffle rhythmically or swirl about in grand ballroom style. It is not even necessary for the penis to be in the vagina for this to be good exercise and great fun.

A second form of coital dancing requires that the man enter the woman from the front or rear while standing. Then they slowly dance. However, the partners must be exactly the correct height in relation to each other so that neither has to stand on tip toe or squat.

You should plan ahead so that you have chosen (or cleared) a spot large enough for dancing. Spontaneity is OK, but you don't want to bump into something or fall, especially if you are naked or coupled. As we have said before, wear a bra or jock if your organs are large, disturb the rhythm or cause bruising.

Any kind of dancing burns calories, so no matter what your age, size or degree of nimbleness, you should consider making it part of Swell-Wimp.[17] It is good for the legs and back and vigorous dancing is good for the cardiovascular system. Wearing heavy footwear burns additional calories, as does wearing a backpack or extra clothing.

SexEx in the Water

Now let's turn our attention to a very different method of increasing energy expenditure during SexAct: SexEx in the water. This can be terrific. You can exercise in any body of water large enough for you to stretch out flat, one foot or more deep and without large waves: large bath tubs, Jacuzzis, hot tubs,[18] ponds, streams, lakes, and even the ocean. Adjust your activities to the site; for example, you can't do sit-ups in a backyard pool five feet deep. Swimming pools are excellent, because in addition to being big enough, they often have steps and grab bars which may be incorporated into the exercises. You must take into account that most pools are treated with chemicals (usually chlorine) which may cause vaginal irritation and you should cease SexExing at the first sign of a problem.

Studies have shown that swimming is one of the best types of exercise: more muscle groups are used than with any other form of exercise[19] and the water helps to keep the body cool and to support your weight (so exercise can continue longer than on land). Thus, pools are good places for large men and women to do Swell-Wimp. The water supports some of their body weight making them feel lighter and enabling them to assume some of the acrobatic positions they can't out of the water. Another benefit is that water provides resistance to movement; the ancient Spartan warriors developed their leg muscles by running through knee-deep water. Finally, psychologically, there is something very pleasant about immersing yourself in water.[20]

In general, water helps to support your body weight, even enabling your limbs to float, so it may take some practice before you can exercise gracefully. For example, sit ups can be awkward at first, because when you lie down your body will tend to float and thus you may tip to the right or left.

You have to learn to work with the supporting water, not against it. For example, leg lifts become leg pulls. Since the water lifts your legs, you have to pull them down instead of lift them up. Attaching water wings to your ankles effectively negates the force of gravity and reverses the action of leg lifts. This gives the muscles in the back of your legs, buttocks and the small of the back a good work out. Push-ups in the water are easier;[21] however, breathing must be regulated carefully since your face will be underwater part of the time.[22]

Knee bends (with the penis in the vagina and the female's legs wrapped around the male's hips) are good in water at least neck-deep (when you are squatting). The water supports the woman's weight at the lower end of the knee bend, but the male bears her full weight when he stands. In deeper water her weight is supported for more of the knee bend, but, of course, both may be under water when he squats.[23] It is difficult, because of anatomy, for the man to enter the woman (front or rear) and clasp her body as she does knee bends. But if your anatomies enable you to do this, then give it a try. Her legs can benefit. Of course, as we said earlier do knee bends with caution since you can injure your knees.

At the deep end of the pool, a couple can do sexual leaps. On the surface the man enters the woman and they wrap their arms around each other. Then they allow themselves to sink to the bottom while remaining vertical. When they reach the bottom, they use their legs to propel themselves back to the surface (leap). Both partners exercise their legs simultaneously and expend considerable energy leaping back to the surface. In addition, this method creates considerable pleasure centered in the groin region, although there is also the possibility of great pain, so be careful.

Because water supports the body's weight, it is easy to do rolls and tumbles. After the man has entered the woman (face-to-face or from the rear), the couple can stretch out and allow themselves to float at the surface. Then they can roll laterally. Or after coupling, they can draw their legs up and tumble head over heels; one partner holds the other while the other uses his or her arms to balance them (keep them on an even keel).

A couple can also swim while coupled. The man enters the woman (face to face) and then they swim about using the side stroke. Each partner uses one arm to stroke and the other to grasp the other. Of course, this cannot be done in a bathtub or Jacuzzi. The water makes the experience more sensual and the swimming burns calories.

Pull ups can be done using a diving board. After the man enters the woman, she wraps her legs around his hips and holds on to his upper body with her arms. The man then pulls them both out of the water by grasping the diving board above his head. Using the same position, the man can wrap his arms around the woman and she can pull them up and down in the water. Pull-ups exercise the shoulder and upper-back muscles but primarily the various muscles of the arms.[24] They are good for burning calories, but they mainly develop muscles that do not have much effect on sexual pleasure. Still, well-developed arm muscles are quickly noticed by others, so doing pull-ups can result in early positive feedback. Further, as your arms get stronger and your body weight declines, pull-ups become easier—another form of positive feedback. Thus, pull-ups are an excellent exercise, especially when done in water.

Sexual exercise completely under water is also very good. Activities take on a wonderful slow-motion aspect. Your lung capacity is developed over a period of time and it may provide you the privacy you desire. Of course, you must be careful; drowning is a very real danger. As we mentioned earlier, a snorkel can be used in many situations. Of course, you may use scuba gear if you own and know how to use it.[25]

Remember that the point is to increase the energy output during lacustrine SexAct. The emphasis should be on integrating sexual activities with exercise in order to burn more calories.

Sex and Cold Temperatures

SexAct in the cold can be especially good, because the body uses energy keeping warm by shivering. Also, goose bumps[26] consume energy, although in minute amounts. You can open windows in the Winter, Spring or Fall if the temperature is below 55 or 60 degrees Fahrenheit and turn up the air-conditioner in the Summer, Spring and Fall so as to keep the bedroom temperature below 60.[27] Kinsey reports that a considerable and developing loss of sensory capacity—including the senses of hearing, smell and taste—begins with sexual arousal and continues to climax.[28] During the earliest phase of SexAct, gentle stroking, rubbing, and caressing stimulate us. The farther along we go, the more it takes to get through to our senses: we become less sensitive to scratching, biting, slapping and other actions that often accompany sexual arousal. After orgasm, sensory perception returns quickly—so much so that touching the penis or clitoris may cause pain. The diminished sensory perception also includes the temperature sense, so you will not feel cold even though your body knows it is cold and works harder to maintain its temperature.

Rubbing cold substances on the body can be effective. Ice, of course, works well, but ice cream and similar things are better, because they smell good and are tasty to remove with the tongue. Ice packs can be placed in the bed or strapped to various parts of the body. However, care must be taken that the sex urge and male erection are not lost due to the cold, so never keep cold substances on the penis, testicles, pudendum, or nipples for too long. Of course, be careful not to injure any tissues due to prolonged exposure to cold and NEVER use dry ice which is frozen carbon dioxide (-110 degrees Fahrenheit) or super-cooled water ice. They actually feel hot to the skin and will always cause injury, often severe.

There are several locations on the body that are especially sensitive to cold and touching them with cold substances immediately results in goose bumps and even shivering (even when the air temperature is quite high). They should be sought out and used at the appropriate times: the area between the second and third toes of each foot; the back of the right knee; the navel; and an area one inch wide and several inches long running from the armpit down the inside of the upper-arm toward the elbow.

Just showering and not wiping off works well, as does wearing wet socks or underwear. Showering together in cold or cool water has two results: calories are expended warming the body and each partner is aroused by the shower and contact with the other. It is generally thought that a cold shower dampens sexual arousal and it can if you shower alone, but showering together is very stimulating unless the water is very cold. Of course, you have to touch (soap, wash, rinse, caress) each other. You can burn many calories by wetting the body (as after a shower) and then engaging in SexAct. Eating cold foods and beverages[29] before SexAct burns calories, because the body must contend with interior and exterior cold.

Since different people respond to cold in different ways, you must experiment. Some people need nothing to make them cold except a room temperature below seventy-five and nakedness. Others will have to leave the windows wide open and probably also employ a fan or ice. Partners with widely differing tolerance to cold should be careful that this does not become a contentious issue between them.

One should never be so cold that shivering interferes with sexual exercise to any significant degree. It should be noted though that the involuntary and semi-involuntary movements associated with shivering can, in fact, enhance the pleasure of sex, often in unpredictable ways; that is, shivering can provide pleasant surprises—also unpleasant ones if the muscle contractions become too violent or occur at the wrong time.

Hot SexEx

SexAct in very warm conditions causes the body to work hard to cool itself. However, with cold SexAct it is easier to regulate the degree of cooling than the degree of warming: you can quickly put on some clothes to warm yourself, but it is more difficult to cool off (you can remove clothing only until you are naked).

Still, you may want to take advantage of hot occasions. For example, when you bake: a hot kitchen makes an excellent location for Swell-Wimp and the smell of the baking bread or pie will enhance your pleasure. You can "turn up the heat" by donning additional clothing (see "Dressing for Swell-Wimp" in Chapter 8), building a fire[30] in the fireplace or by using hand and foot warmers such as those used by hunters.

SexEx Outdoors

All of the preceding exercises can be done outdoors—"Amang the rigs o'barley" as Robert Burns says. Choose your location carefully: you don't want to be disturbed by flies, ants, snakes, little children, opossums, dogs, armadillos, street vendors, scorpions or deer.[31] Sex outdoors can add an element of "naughtiness" that many people find arousing, but it can also add a certain element of illegality depending upon where you exercise. Certainly in front of the court house is not a good place. Not even all nude beaches are acceptable because any activity that can be construed as sexual can be deemed illegal. So check local rules and regulations before you exercise. Even your own backyard might not be safe if your neighbors can see you and complain that you are engaging in public lewdness. Rooftops with fencing are almost perfect since it is unlikely that anyone can look down upon or up at you. However, the Supreme Court upheld a state law forbidding sodomy even between married couples in the privacy of their own homes. And these older, heterosexual males (primarily) also held that new evidence of innocence is not grounds for a new trial after a specified time. That is, you are innocent until proven guilty and nevermore. Therefore, the privacy of your own fenced rooftop might not keep you out of trouble.

Still, it is often much simpler (and cheaper) to go outside for SexEx than to turn up the heat or turn on the air-conditioner. SexEx outdoors at night under the stars and in the moonlight is tremendously romantic.

The chemical that produces the pollen-like odor of fresh semen (which is a mild aphrodisiac) is contained in thalictrum flowers and is released when grass is cut. Many, if not most, people are "turned on" by freshly mown grass. This is another reason you might want to consider SexEx outdoors—near a golf course, cemetery, ball field or even in the back yard.

Because of the diminished sensory sensitivity that accompanies sexual arousal, you must be careful to avoid sunburn and frost bite, especially of sensitive areas, such as the penis and nipples. And because SexEx is so much fun, you must take precautions to avoid heat stroke since you may disregard its symptoms as simply physiological changes due to arousal.[32] We recommend that you—even you sun lovers—always perform SexEx in the shade;[33] this will help prevent overheating and burning of sensitive body parts and possibly hide you from the notice of others.

Conclusion

The aim of the techniques in this chapter is to burn additional calories and thus lose weight and strengthen muscles. The point is not to impress your partner(s) with the number of sit-ups or leg lifts you can do. Also, keep in mind that when you first begin to exercise, your muscles may feel tight and sore. With the abdominal muscles, this will result in a feeling that you cannot stand up straight (and, in fact, it may be difficult for you to do so). You may want to begin new exercises on Friday night so that the soreness will have worn off before you have to go to work on Monday.

Every physical activity burns calories. Moving large parts of the body (leg lifts) uses more energy than moving small parts (blinking), but any movement uses some.

So the partner doing leg lifts, sit-ups or pushups is burning a lot of calories. The other partner can too. He or she should not just sit (or lie) there. "Inactive" partners can do head rolls, windmills with the arms, neck arches, and so on. He or she can also employ the techniques that were described in Chapter 6—sing, yell, tell jokes and so on.[34] Just as there is no "passive" partner during good sex, there is no "passive" partner during Swell-Wimp.

It is important of remember that the primary aim of SexAct is pleasure. What we have described in this chapter are techniques that can be used to increase caloric expenditure during SexAct. These should not be allowed to interfere with sexual pleasure.[35] Swell-Wimp should not be like low-calorie cream puffs, which are so little like real cream puffs that they are not worth eating. SexEx should not be so little like real SexAct that it is not worth doing. Most of our study subjects found that they could include the techniques into SexAct easily and quickly. And several found that they actually enhanced SexAct: they found it more interesting, exciting and fulfilling. Some of the techniques were actually developed by the study subjects, so experiment. Develop your own techniques. As Friedrich Nietzsche says, "One repays a teacher badly if one always remains nothing but a pupil."[36]

Chapter 11

Postplay

Postplay is not given much attention by researchers, writers or sexual partners. Comedians make jokes about how women like to cuddle and talk after intercourse and men just want to go to sleep. But postplay is no joke. There is some evidence that the high rate of heart attack in men may be due, in part, to the fact that they neglect postplay.[1] Since SexAct is physical exercise, SexExers need to "cool down" just as runners continue to jog slowly after a race. Postplay helps to prevent cramping because waste products are eliminated from the muscles. Respiration and heart rates are slowed gradually. The body switches from maximum cooling (profuse sweating) to normal cooling or even back to heating.

Kinsey reports that after orgasm, sensory perception returns very quickly—so much so that some men experience pain if the penis is touched. And Shere Hite reports that there are some women who are unable to experience multiple orgasms because their clitorises become too sensitive to touch after the first. Both females and males may feel "itchy" and need to urinate. Many people experience "post coitum triste" (after coitus one is sad), a feeling of quiescence and calmness rather than sadness. Some are ready in a few minutes to resume normal activities but others fall asleep.

After orgasm, men return physiologically to the pre-arousal state. Women, on the other hand, return to the pre-orgasmic plateau and then slowly return to the pre-arousal state. That is, after orgasm, men are back where they started (limp penis and all) except that they have experienced an episode of sexual satisfaction. Women return to where they were before orgasm; having experienced sexual satisfaction, they are still aroused and ready to achieve orgasm again.[2] Shere Hite reports that after orgasm most women (1) feel tender and loving and want to be close to their partners and (2) strong and wide awake.[3] Thus, postplay should take a different course for males and females. The male simply needs to "cool off" physiologically, whereas the female needs emotional/psychological as well as physiological cooling off. This means the male should, at least, not just roll over and go to sleep, but snuggle and caress his partner for a while.

Cooling Down

Think of the body during sex as a car traveling down the road at 55 miles per hour. During orgasm you zoom to 120 mph. If you slam on the brakes, throw the transmission into park, shut off the ignition and jump out, you are going to damage something. The same is true of the human body. It is a marvelous thing, but it is better able to go quickly from 0 to 55, than from 55 to 0.[4]

This is an aspect of being human left over from our earliest days. In stressful situations, hormones are dumped into the blood stream and within seconds our hearts are pumping quickly, our breathing is accelerated, our muscles are tensed and we are ready to fight a saber-toothed tiger (or run away).

This is not much use today, unless you are regularly involved in life-threatening situations (police, fire fighters, teachers). For most of us, this atavistic response is a detriment. The supervisor asks us to come to the office and within seconds we become sweating, panting animals (because of the flight-or-fight reaction); we are afraid of what he or she will say. Incidentally there is also evidence that certain categories of persons, such as police, fire fighters and teachers, suffer higher rates of heart disease because they regularly are involved in flight-or-fight situations without the benefit of sufficient cool-down periods.

So what should you do after SexAct? Well it's not so much what you do; just do something sensible and moderate. If your SexAct has been accompanied by music, you should switch to something slower and more restful, such as John Cage's *4' 33''*. You may want to continue caressing, kissing and nibbling. Or you can get up and walk around for a while. If you have been using the techniques for increasing energy expenditure discussed in the previous chapters, you should gently continue with the technique for a short time. For example, if you have been doing sexual sit-ups, do a few more, slowly, to allow the stomach muscles to rid themselves of waste products.

Don'ts

There are some things you should not do during postplay. The genitalia of many men and women become very sensitive after orgasm, so touching them can become painful. Further, their surfaces have been rubbed, bumped, sucked, and tickled; they need time to recover. Take your cue from your partner; if there is any indication that he or she is not enjoying continued genital caressing, stop immediately. You should not eat immediately after SexAct; this draws the blood to the digestive system and away from the muscles and other organs that need the blood to bring oxygen and nutrients and to carry away waste products. Do not engage in strenuous exercise for the same reason and because you may overwork muscles and organs that need rest.[5] Wait a while to take a cold or hot shower or bath. After orgasm, the skin is very sensitive and susceptible to injury. Further, hot and cold temperatures force the body to divert energy to cooling and heating. This might seem like a good idea since it burns calories, but it diverts energy resources away from the more immediate and necessary need for muscle and organ recovery.

Dos

We recommend the following as a model for postplay. After climax, if you have been doing sexual exercises, do several more. Take a few moments to bask in the glow, gently caressing your partner and talking.[6] Micturate if necessary. Depending upon where you are and how strenuous your SexAct was, you may want to shower in warm water. At least, wash your face, hands and genitalia in warm water and gently dry with a soft towel. Pick up the tissues[7] and clothing off the floor. Straighten any furniture you have knocked over and put away any special clothing, equipment and other paraphernalia you have been using. Have a drink of a lukewarm beverage to replenish lost fluids. Avoid depressants (alcohol) and stimulants (coffee) at this time. If you have worked up an appetite have a snack, such as the low-calorie, Italian "desserts" fantoccini and stanlitucci; both provide bulk which ameliorates hunger.

Then, depending upon your situation, do what you normally would. You may prepare for sleep (brush or remove your teeth,[8] take your medication, put on your night clothes, put out the cat, and so on) or dress to go (or return) to work or home or wherever. This will allow your body to slow down while continuing to burn some calories. If you simply go to sleep after SexAct, you will stop expending energy and you risk injury.

Chapter 12

Food and Diet

We become overweight because we take in more calories than we use. As we have pointed out, you can lose weight by burning more calories (Swell-Wimp) or taking in fewer. We will not say much here about diet, because the emphasis of this book is on increasing caloric expenditure through SexEx and because you can obtain good information about dieting from many sources. There are, however, some points we feel compelled to make.

You should avoid sexual bulimia. That is, don't binge eat and then try to engage in SexEx to burn the calories. You probably can't have that much sex without hurting your and your partner's sexual apparatus. As we have said before, you should practice moderation in all things—food, exercise, work, leisure and sex.

Balanced Diet

Eating is a sensory experience—taste and smell and sight and feel.[1] Many people are overweight because they get immediate pleasure from eating; it is the one good thing that they can count on—at least to smell or taste good. Most of the time, overeating is a psychological disorder (there are very few people who really have a "glandular problem"). Further, overeating can become habitual like smoking. Add to this the barrage of advertisements for food and drink that we are subjected to daily. Thus, overeating is the result of a complex of factors that disrupt good eating habits. So, in order to lose weight, you must have the will power to control your diet.

Any diet is acceptable—macrobiotic, vegetarian, or whatever—as long as you get enough nutrients and avoid extremes of fats, sugars, and other "bad" things. You do not have to eat six-course meals; you can often get adequate nutrition from a single dish made of several ingredients, such as New York salmagundi, French ragout, British stews, Menippean satura, and Spanish olio.

You should, of course, follow your physician's instructions concerning diet, if you have any condition, such as diabetes or high blood pressure, that warrants special dieting. Generally, you can't go wrong selecting foods from the four food groups (as we have been taught since grade school). For example, you might choose yogurt from the dairy group, spinach from the vegetable group, pumpernickel from the cereals group and chicken wings from the meat group. Add to this a beverage[2] and a dessert[3] and you have a nutritious, delicious balanced meal that will provide the energy for SexEx.[4]

Quick Energy

Some foods deliver energy quickly; the energy (primarily sugars) enters the blood stream and is delivered to the muscles quickly. These are good before or during SexAct for a quick energy boost. Athletes often use them. Especially good is the French *pastiche y melange* (pasta and melon) which contains both carbohydrates and quick-energy sugars. Glorp, the high-energy mixture used by mountain climbers, is a good choice as are the various "trail mixes" used by hikers. They provide long-term energy. You can keep some by the side of your bed and "snack" during an extended SexAct session.

After SexAct you should replenish your energy stores and satisfy the hunger that exercise often stimulates. Choose some of the same low-calorie and quick-energy foods that you eat before SexAct.

Aphrodisiacs

An aphrodisiac is a substance that stimulates or intensifies sexual desire and pleasure, whether eaten, drunk, inhaled, rubbed on the body, or injected. Such substances do exist, but there is much misinformation about them. Since Swell-Wimp is designed to be easy and natural (as well as fun), the use of aphrodisiacs is not necessary or recommended.

The most famous aphrodisiac is probably "Spanish fly." It is made from (Spanish) beetles which are dried, pulverized and treated in order to extract a substance called cantharidin, which is tremendously irritating. When it is ingested and then excreted (urination), it stimulates the sex organs by irritating them, causing mild to extreme discomfort. It does not increase sexual desire but may intensify sexual pleasure by sensitizing the genitalia. Cantharidin is toxic to humans and even a little bit too much can cause death. Spanish fly should be avoided; the risks far outweigh the dubious benefits.

Eating "prairie oysters" (bull's testicles) was advocated in the nineteenth century. They have to be eaten raw and fresh, and even then most of the male sex hormone is destroyed by the digestive process. We do not recommend them; they are expensive, difficult to obtain fresh and really don't do much.

There are some aphrodisiac drugs. Strychnine (also called "nux vomica") sensitizes the nervous system and thus it can increase response to sexual stimulation, but only when taken in very minute amounts; otherwise, it causes death by convulsions. Do not use it! The famous Yohimbine, made from the inner bark of an African tree, doesn't work. Marijuana is reported to cause sexual arousal, sexual fantasies, and increased sexual sensation but it is illegal. For some people, the purchase and use of marijuana—the illegal activity—turns them on, not the drug itself. However, being arrested is generally a turn off, so do not use it. David Reuben says that LSD is a powerful aphrodisiac for some people.[5] However, for other people it is a mind-destroyer! It is a controlled-substance and, therefore, illegal. It is much too dangerous to fool around with.

Testosterone, the male sex hormone, is a true aphrodisiac; it causes powerful sexual desire in men and women. However, it cannot be obtained legally; it causes atrophy of the testicles in men and masculinization in women; it provokes aggressive behavior; and it causes liver damage in both sexes. The price of using testosterone is too high.

Alcohol is not a true aphrodisiac. Because it is a "downer," it can reduce fear, tension and anxiety which interfere with sexual stimulation. Further, it can decrease inhibitions. Thus, it can make a sexual encounter easier, especially if you fear failure.[6] But it interferes with coordination and diminishes sensation, so it lessens sexual pleasure. And a lack of inhibitions and a diminished sense of fear can have disastrous results! We recommend that you avoid alcoholic beverages as much as possible, especially in connection with SexAct. If you don't need it to overcome fear, it will lessen your pleasure and if you do need it to overcome fear or anxiety, you should do something about this problem and not rely on alcohol. Besides, alcoholic beverages are high in calories and thus they work against weight loss.

Chilies contain capsicin which drives the nervous system crazy; so the brain floods the nerve endings with endorphins which are the body's natural painkillers.[7] Thus, after you eat some chili (after the "chili sweat"), it doesn't seem as hot and you start to feel good. A chili high is like a runner's high; it is the result of the endorphins. Although chilies are not aphrodisiacs, orgasm combined with a chili high is an interesting experience.

Some foods, such as oysters, eggs, clams, onions, celery, sausages, and asparagus, resemble the sex organs, but they have no aphrodisiac powers despite what you may have heard or read. Like ginseng and rhinoceros horn, they "work" because the user wants them to work.[8] The most powerful sex organ is the brain. If the brain believes that eating wieners will increase sexual desire, then it probably will.[9] The best aphrodisiacs are those that stimulate the nerve receptors of the sexually sensitive parts of the body (rubbing, licking, kissing) and the brain, which is accessed through the eyes, ears, nose and tongue.

Fluids

You should drink plenty of liquids during SexAct in order to replenish those lost through ejaculation, sweating, lushing,[10] weeping, and drooling. You may want to keep a carafe of Gatorade or even plain water near-by.[11] Of course, you should avoid beverages high in calories (soft drinks, Kool-Aid, fruit juices). Don't drink too much because this can interfere with sexual enjoyment (running to the bathroom) or cause distress (coitus with a full bladder). Our study has shown that it is very rare indeed that enough fluids are lost to warrant taking salt tablets, although there was one intense weekend in August when, as a precaution, all four participants asked for some. Of course, avoid alcoholic beverages which are high in calories and suppress the sex drive.[12]

It should be noted that human semen is a nutritious substance. Although it is high in sugar (glucose) and contains some salts and cholesterol, it also contains calcium, protein and carbohydrates. Thus, those who engage in fellatio, in addition to making themselves and their partners feel good and in addition to expending energy, also take in (if they ingest) a small amount of nutritious substance, thereby replenishing lost calories (glucose is immediately changed to energy) resulting in more energy for continued exercise. This is more enjoyable than eating a candy bar.

However, semen is slightly acidic and may have a lightly bitter taste (depending upon the amount of urea in it); *degustibus non est disputandum*—it is an acquired taste. NOTE: you should not attempt to meet your daily dietary requirements by ingesting only semen (either by repeated fellatio or by saving it). Semen does NOT contain a number of vitamins and minerals and will not provide a balanced diet by itself. Further, ingesting semen can be dangerous. Since AIDS is transmitted via bodily fluids, you must be careful when engaging in fellatio (and cunnilingus). You can reduce your chances of infection by not swallowing the semen, by using some sort of protection (such as a condom), and by exercising only with a long-time partner. We cannot tell you not to engage in oral sex, but you should be VERY careful.

After SexAct you will almost certainly be thirsty. Watermelon is good for cooling down and replacing lost fluids. It is a deliciously red, juicy, inexpensive, low-calorie food. A small, uncut watermelon, smooth and round, is wonderfully pleasing to the eye as you open the refrigerator door and the cool air wafts over your sweaty body. It is also nice to put one on the night stand or dresser—whole or sliced to expose the interior—where you can see it during SexAct. In fact, you might want to make up a fruit bowl of melons, cherries and bananas to place on the night stand.

Snacking

As everyone knows, snacking is not healthful. Snack foods are usually high in fats, carbohydrates, and salt; they are full of empty calories. They cause our appetites to decrease, so we eat fewer of the good foods at meal time. Thus, snacking must be avoided if you want to lose or maintain your weight. But it is hard to break old eating habits. What can you do?

We recommend that when you get the urge for a Danish, buttered buns, potato chips or even a beer, you engage in SexAct instead. It's pleasurable, it burns calories and it will help break the snacking habit. When you first begin Swell-Wimp, you will probably have been snacking frequently, so you should develop a brief SexEx to substitute for snacking. You should be able to begin and finish quickly; if you try to substitute a major exercise, you will most likely return to snacking because the pleasure is more immediate (or you will find yourself almost continually engaged in SexEx).

It seems probable to us that a brief SexEx could also be used to break the smoking habit. When you get the urge to light up, you could just lie down. We must point out that we can find no studies concerning this and that we have not as yet been able to conduct such a study.[13] If you smoke a lot, you might want to substitute SexAct for every other or every third cigarette, because engaging in SexAct thirty to forty times a day may be too much—physically and psychologically.

Food-Flavored and Food-Scented Products

The part of the brain that reacts to smells, the rhinecephalon, is a very primitive apparatus, a vestige from our earliest times as living organisms. Even though the modern human sense of smell is greatly diminished (we depend much more upon sight), smells affect us in a primitive and powerful way. The links between smells and times, places and activities are strong and apparently permanent. Thus, the tiniest whiff of an odor can evoke distant memories or fill us with disgust, and the smell of a favorite food can make us ravenously hungry in a way that a morning's hard work does not; this is called the Zibeta Occidentalis effect. Since the purpose of Swell-Wimp is to maintain or lose weight, you do not want to work against this purpose by filling your SexEx environment with smells that will cause you to eat.[14] However, you can take advantage of this phenomenon by introducing smells into your "bedroom" that arouse you. For example, some people are turned on by the smell of crisp new money, although as even the Romans knew, *pecunia non olet*.[15]

When you begin Swell-Wimp, you should avoid food-flavored and food-scented shampoos, creams, unguents, and so on. The intimacy of sexual exercise will bring you into close contact with them, which will remind you of the pleasures of eating and rouse your appetite. Of course, avoid any use of honey,[16] chocolate syrup, peanut butter and any similar foods during sexual activity. They can heighten sexual pleasure (spread them on the penis or vagina before fellatio or cunnilingus), but contain many calories. We recommend that you find low-calorie substitutes, such as "lite" pancake syrup, low-calorie fruit juices and beef bouillon.[17]

If your weight is correct and your Swell-Wimp is designed to keep you fit, then you may indulge yourself, but be moderate. Licking an entire can of chocolate syrup from your partner's body can be just as bad as (although more fun than) eating a handful of candy bars. Using food in moderation as part of your sexual exercise can be very pleasurable, since you combine sexual and gustatory pleasure with the psychological pleasure derived from the knowledge that you are doing good things for your body.

Other Uses of Food

Foods can be chosen for more than their nutritional value. There are many wholesome foods, so you may also select for other reasons, such as sensory appeal (pleasing to taste, look at or smell), stimulative value (red, juicy, hard), and even aphrodisiac power. Why eat corn when you can eat something more suggestive, such as Brussels sprouts, melon halves or asparagus?

Because food is more than an experience of taste, it can be used in other ways. That is, looking at, smelling and feeling some foods can be pleasurable.[18] You may want to use food decoratively. As mentioned before, you can place a fruit bowl in the bedroom. Bananas, cherries and melons are suggestive and smell good. There may be smells that you find especially pleasurable or even arousing.[19] For example, you might sprinkle bacon bits or spermicelli about the room if they arouse you but don't make you hungry.

Quod cibus est aliis, aliis est venum.[20] There are a number of phallic and yonic[21] plants that are not good to eat, but which you may want to use to decorate your bedroom, van, or wherever. For example, the Yellow Calla Lily (zantedeschia elliottiana) is tubular with a phallic center. Many orchids are yonic. The mushroom, Cornucopia Craterellus (Craterellus cornucopioides) is yonic and Geaster hygrometricus is breast-like. Mushrooms and fungus, such as Morchella bispora, the "Lord of Erection" toadstool, and Ithyphallus impudicus (especially), some stinkhorns like Dictyophora ravenelli, and even cattail heads, are phallic. And, of course, there are bananas, cucumbers and Marvel's melon. The long, ornamental Peter pepper, known to some botanists as the "penis pepper," makes an excellent decoration for the bedroom, especially if you are into New Mexican cuisine and lifestyles; it just fits in so well.

The association of the smell of foods that you especially like with sexual pleasure can help you to lose weight—a kind of smell therapy. Rather than associating the smell of pork chops, French fries or cream puffs with their taste and the feeling of fullness you get when you eat them, you will associate them with sexual pleasure. You will not want to immediately eat them; instead you will become aroused and want to engage in SexAct—which burns calories! We see no danger that the olfactory links will become so strong that you will become unduly aroused when you go near a Burger King. It is more likely that when you smell French fries, you will not immediately want some but will think in terms of "Where is she (he) now?" If you can't get to your partner, you will smile and know that you do not have to gorge yourself on French fries, but will satisfy yourself later in a different more healthy manner.

Alex Comfort's *The New Joy of Sex* is subtitled *A Gourmet Guide to Lovemaking for the Nineties*. Throughout he uses the metaphor that making love is like cooking—gourmet cooking—and the section titles refer to main courses, sauces, and so on. This is an excellent book but his view is diametrically opposed to ours. SexAct is not cordon bleu cooking. To us, it is whole grains and vegetables with fruits and honey for dessert—natural and wholesome, not rich and fattening. We cannot live on sauces and relishes alone. Basic foods and SexEx in moderate amounts result in pleasurable healthfulness.

Chapter 13

Equipment

Alex Comfort claims that an Austrian gymnastic professor, Van Weck Erlen, wrote a book advocating sexual activity as part of a general physical fitness lifestyle (Turnergesellschaft). Apparently, Erlen described a "sexuarium" complete with mats, trapezes, mirrors, red light and black decor.[1] We are unfamiliar with Erlen's "sexuarium," but we know lots of people who think that in order to lose weight you must use exercise equipment. One of the major advantages of Swell-Wimp is that it does not require special gear. You can integrate Swell-Wimp with some kinds of exercise paraphernalia but you do not have to purchase jogging outfits, rowing machines, special shoes, bicycles, or weights. Nor do you have to purchase food scales or special record-keeping journals. Swell-Wimp is natural and can be done almost anywhere, anytime. Still, there are some pieces of equipment you may want to use or obtain.

Take Precautions

The first and most important item is some method of birth control (see Chapter 9). Since Swell-Wimp[2] is based upon frequent SexAct, you must take steps to prevent an unwanted flower in your apron. The method you choose is, of course, up to you. If you have decided you don't want any (more) children, then avoid the continuing cost of birth control and have yourself permanently sterilized.

If you are less than eighteen years of age, you should seriously consider remaining celibate until you are. In some neighborhoods where drug use is common, complete abstinence is the only way to avoid sexual-related AIDS infection. Clearly, we advocate frequent SexAct for weight loss and maintenance, but for some people in some situations in some places, abstention is a sensible choice.

Unless you ALWAYS engage in SexAct with the same partner, you (male or female) should carry condoms at all times and USE THEM. AIDS is no joke and currently condoms are the only device that demonstrates any effectiveness in preventing infection.[3] Even if you have had a long-term sexual relationship with a single partner, you may want to consider using condoms, unless you are absolutely sure of the nature of your partner's sex life before your relationship began and you are absolutely sure that he or she is not having sexual relations with anyone else.[4] Condoms are not a fail-safe prophylactic against AIDS, but they do provide some protection and they are cheap and easy to carry. Don't leave home without them.

Home-Exercise Equipment

According to the January 1998 issue of *Consumer Reports* (63: 1), home exercise equipment is both expensive and unreliable and it takes up a lot of room. Further, "[m]ost of our testers found using riders and walkers monotonous" (28). We believe that this is true of using most if not all exercise equipment. Remaining rooted to a spot in a room and doing monotonous repetitive activity used to be called work; today, people willingly pay money to do this. We simply find it absurd to purchase and use contraptions costing from $900 to $2500 for exercising instead of doing something useful (picking up trash along the highway, gardening, cutting wood, or painting the house) or interesting (playing tennis, basketball, or tag) or pleasurable (Swell-Wimp).

Only a very small part of the population actually needs home-exercise equipment: those who for some medical condition must exercise a particular part of the body or are not ambulatory enough for more sensible exercise; those who cannot leave home (under house arrest, for example); those such as lawyers and legislators who are unable to engage in any activities (such as team sports) in which they are not the center of attention; and public-school teachers (who teach all day, grade papers and prepare lessons at night and on the weekends in addition to supervising extra-curricular activities and taking care of their own families; they often can exercise only for half an hour or so after the kids have been put to bed).[5]

Our studies have shown that you shouldn't try Swell-Wimp on exercise bikes, cross-country ski machines, walkers, riders, or elliptical exercisers. (We discuss using stationary bikes and rowing-machines for warming up in Chapter 5). You may want to try Swell-Wimp on a rowing machine or stair climber but you should be careful and dexterous: we leave it to your imagination.

Swell-Wimp does integrate well with treadmills which "have long been the best-selling exercise machine in the U.S.—Americans spent $1.4 billion on treadmills in 1996" (*Consumer Reports*, Jan 1998, 22). First, a treadmill can be used for warming up. Most can accommodate two people who can run (naked), rubbing and bumping into each other. Or one person can carry the other (both naked, of course) and jog at a slow speed. Then the other person carries the first person and jogs. However, the best use of a treadmill for Swell-Wimp is to turn the motor off and use the running platform (cushioned by a pad or blanket) as your Swell-Wimp bed (maybe after you have warmed up with a jog). With all but the cheapest treadmills, the angle of incli-nation of the running bed can be changed by the push of a button. Using this facility during Swell Wimp can enhance your pleasure and cause you to expend more calo-ries (in effect, have sex on a hill). As everyone knows doing anything on a hill requires more energy than on level ground. Many treadmills give you the ability to program the course you run (or use pre-programmed courses); that is, the treadmill automatically changes the running bed's angle, simulating hills and level ground, so you don't even have to think about this during Swell Wimp. Also most treadmills have a pulse sensor built in (a head band or chest strap is preferable to a thumb sen-sor); monitoring their heart rates is important to some Swell Wimpers.

As you can see Swell-Wimp and treadmills integrate well and if you have a tread-mill, by all means, try it. But we don't recommend that you purchase one specifi-cally for Swell-Wimp. You can simulate this form of energy-intensive Swell Wimp by simply placing blocks under one end of your bed or by Swell-Wimping on a hilly part of a lawn.

The Bed

For most people, a bed is a necessary piece of equipment, but a proper Swell-Wimp regime must be flexible, so you must be prepared for SexEx wherever and whenever the opportunity arises. A firm mattress is better than a soft one,[6] but a big bed is not necessarily better than a small one, which can create an intimacy not avail-able in a large bed.[7] Further, SexEx in a small bed can expend extra calories because you have to move about more frequently just to establish and maintain positions. Choose the bed carefully, since you will be spending a considerable amount of time in it (if you are serious about Swell-Wimp).[8] Some people like beds with tall, phallic, corner posts while others prefer round beds.

SexAct on a water bed is different from, not better or worse than, SexAct on a regular bed; it is an acquired taste.[9] They are heavier and more expensive than regular beds and require more maintenance. Those who have mastered coitus on a water bed say there is nothing like it (your body's movements must synchronize with the wave-like motions of the bed). However, some people have been injured when their violent orgasmic motions synchronized with the waves of the water-filled mattress and they were tossed on the floor.

If you have a back problem (see Chapter 8), you may want to consider using a padded exercise mat like those used for wrestling and gymnastics. They provide a firm but not hard platform for SexAct. The smaller ones can be slid beneath your bed or rolled up in a closet when not in use. They are also excellent for carrying in the trunk of your car or in the back of your van. Do not use an air mattress because it does not provide firm support; in fact, because most are ribbed, it is easy to fall off (which is not conducive to orgasm). Further, having to blow a mattress up can delay SexEx, although it does expend quite a bit of energy. They are also much cheaper than padded mats. So if you do not have a back problem and do have good balance, you might want to consider an air mattress. Keep in mind that a carpeted floor is as good as a bed for most SexEx.

Of course, you can have two beds—one with a soft mattress for sleeping and one with a firm mattress for SexAct. However, most bedrooms are not large enough to accommodate two beds, so we recommend two bedrooms—one a traditional bedroom and the other furnished primarily for SexEx (see "The Ideal Bedroom" later in this chapter). If the "sex bed" is put in a different room, you must take care not to separate the intimacy of arousal, cuddling and sleeping from SexAct; you should never hesitate to engage in SexAct in the traditional bedroom nor sleep in the SexEx bedroom. Still, most people do not have an extra bedroom[10] and having two bedrooms runs counter to the Swell-Wimp philosophy—easy, natural, fun and inexpensive.

The top of the mattress should be level with the man's pubic bone for access from the side. Generally, cheaper beds are quite low and make it difficult to use any of the positions for SexEx in which one partner stands on the floor and the other reclines on the bed. In the long run it is worth the trouble and expense of finding a bed of the right height.[11]

Miscellaneous Items

You should have a cloth towel, handkerchief, roll of paper towels, box of wet wipes or something similar to clean up with.[12] Always properly dispose of them; do not throw them out of the car window or leave them laying under a bush or on the floor for the maid to pick up. It is incumbent upon each one of us in every facet of our lives to take care of the environment.[13]

If you will be engaging in SexAct outdoors, you should carry a blanket or a piece of plastic sheeting (it requires little room when folded) to lay on. Carry it with you also if you will be engaging in SexAct indoors, but cannot predict the location beforehand (in the office, kitchen, warehouse, garage, gymnasium). Or you can carry a small air mattress that can be filled quickly with a CO_2 cartridge.

You may want (or need) to monitor your physical condition or progress during sexual activity. A pedometer can be attached to the hip (modify a garter belt with Velcro) to keep track of the number of thrusts. If necessary, keep a watch and stethoscope by the bedside. You should attach a sphygmomanometer cuff before starting SexAct, if your condition warrants.

A metronome can be a useful piece of equipment, especially if you vocalize during SexEx. Begin at a nice Largo (42) and increase the setting during SexEx or set it to a higher setting at the beginning of each session. If you can exercise at Allegro settings of 170 or higher, sexual exercise will become truly aerobic as your heart and respiration rates reach those of competitive athletes. On the other hand, with experimentation you can find a rate slow enough to keep you exercising for long periods of time without climaxing and the longer you exercise the more calories you burn.

You should also have readily at hand any other things you like or need, such as your favorite pillow, comedy albums, lubricants, identification, ankle weights, a fan, special clothing, and so on.

If your SexEx location changes frequently, you should purchase a large purse, briefcase, book bag, or back pack to carry the equipment. If you often engage in SexAct in your car or van,[14] you can keep most your "equipment" there, but you should still carry your birth control device and/or condoms on your person. Incidentally, an automobile is a good site for SexEx because the size of the interior forces you to try new positions and to frequently adjust position to avoid cramps. This results in more calories being expended and can help you become more limber and flexible. You should, of course, be careful because it is easy to injure yourself in an automobile; there are many sharp edges and protrusions such as the gear shift and turn signal levers.[15]

Most "sex manuals" devote a number of pages to intercourse on swings—garden swings, porch swings, hanging-basket swings, and so on. The swooping motion of the swing results in an alternation of negative and positive G-forces which pleasurably stimulates the sex organs. We do not advocate the use of swings for Swell-Wimp. SexEx on a swing does not burn additional calories. If you use an outdoor swing, you will encounter all of the problems associated with outdoor SexEx—bugs, heat, cold, sunburn, voyeurs, irate neighbors and so on. An indoor swing requires a lot of room and can be quite expensive. Further, many of you are beginning Swell-Wimp because you are obese. Attempting Swell-Wimp on a swing will only make it more difficult for you without resulting in an appreciable increase in energy expenditure. Whether you are overweight or not, the risk of injury is substantial. All of these objections apply equally to SexEx in small boats and canoes. Engaging in SexAct on a swing or in a boat has a nice romantic quality about it, but Swell-Wimp is not about romance; it's about burning up a maximum number of calories in a natural and inexpensive manner through sexual activity.[16]

Interruptions

There is another piece of equipment that most people would not associate with SexAct, but which we rank as essential—the telephone answering machine. The ringing of a telephone can cause an erect penis to droop and bring SexEx to a halt. Many people can talk on the phone and get dressed, cook supper, continue to work, or watch TV. But very few people can talk on the phone and engage in SexAct at the same time.[17] When you are climbing up the mountain toward orgasm, you cannot simply stop for a while to answer the phone. If you do, you will slide all or most of the way back to the bottom. An answering machine can let you continue the climb.

Unfortunately, even the sound of a telephone ringing can be disruptive. It is a sudden unpleasant sound. Whether the phone has an old-fashioned bell or a modern electronic ringer, it is meant to call attention to itself. Even if you don't have to answer the phone, the ringing of the bell can interrupt SexAct. This does not mean that you are in any way deficient, not a real man or woman. A backfire or car horn, the doorbell, the sound of something being dropped—any sudden and less-than-pleasant sound can interrupt SexAct. Also, we grow up thinking that the phone MUST be answered (even though we know that most of the time the call could wait).[18] So turn off your phone or turn down the ringer's volume (or put it in a drawer if you can) and turn on the answering machine.

Don't think that you are unlikely to be interrupted by the phone. If fact, if you usually don't get many phone calls, the ringing will be even more disruptive. You may think that since you only get a call from someone (your mom, kids, ex-spouse) once-a-week, the phone won't be a problem, but today's computer-assisted direct-marketing organizations call tens of thousands of people at all times, day and night. What could be worse than being about to culminate a pleasant and energy-intensive SexEx in orgasm, and having to answer the phone and listen to a computer-generated voice try to sell you insurance or have the person at the other end of the line ask "Who's this?"[19] And, living in the "boondocks" is no protection.

Statistically, you are much more likely to be interrupted by a telephone call than by someone at the door. However, if you live where people frequently come to the door, you may want to consider installing a switch on the doorbell so it can be turned off. Unfortunately, there is not much you can do to prevent people from knocking. Don't post a message that says you are not at home; this is an open invitation to burglars. You may want to consider finding a different location for SexEx. If you are in a hotel, you can hang a "Do not disturb" sign, but sometimes this doesn't work either.[20]

Pets can also interrupt SexEx; they can jump on the bed, scratch at the door, whine and howl. You should feed them and let them "do their business" (if they do it outside) before you begin. And, of course, you should wind the clock BEFORE you begin.

Incidentally, if you are very isolated geographically or home-bound or if for some other reason your primary sexual outlet takes place via the telephone, you can integrate Swell-Wimp with "phone sex." However, it should be obvious that "phone sex," even via 900 telephone numbers, will probably not result in much weight loss. We hope to address this issue in our studies of auto-erotic Swell-Wimp, when funding becomes available. In the meantime you might want to read Nicholson Baker's book *Vox* on this subject.[21]

Vans

Several times we have mentioned using a van for SexEx. A van enables you to get away from the phone, work, kids, parents, relatives, and a myriad of other problems and distractions. Using a van may be the only way that some people can do Swell-Wimp and for others it can add the spice that makes SexEx attractive. Most of us settle into a routine, engaging in SexAct at the same times and places because of work, family and other obligations. Choosing other times and places can add vigor and spice to your sex life and even reawaken sleeping interest.

Of course, driving to some safe, convenient and pleasant location does eliminate spontaneity, but it may be the only way. Having your own van can be more convenient than traveling to a motel or hotel and in the long run it may be cheaper. If you own a van, try it. Otherwise, we don't recommend purchasing one; they are expensive and may just sit in the driveway unused like the exercise equipment in the basement. However, the adventure of SexEx in a van may be the factor that finally gets you to try Swell-Wimp; you may be just too lazy, complacent, stubborn or apathetic to try other methods of exercise.[22]

There is another factor in favor of SexEx in a van: you can travel to different locations. Each session can take place in a different environment with new sights and sounds. You do, however, have to be wary of voyeurs, police officers, and trouble makers. Be aware that SexEx in a van (or car) can raise the humidity quite high; leave a window partially open.

The Ideal Bedroom

If you always engage in SexEx at the same location, you can "equip" it for maximum energy expenditure and pleasure. Sexual orgasm is primarily physiological; a paralyzed person can achieve orgasm. But sexual arousal is primarily psychological. Thus, your SexEx location should be equipped and decorated for maximum arousal for you and your partner(s).[23] Anything that may interfere with arousal and efficient and pleasurable SexEx should be eliminated.

Let's assume that you will be using your bedroom at home. First, choose the appropriate type of bed or mat. Depending upon your preference, install an air conditioner or a heater to raise or lower the temperature for maximum calorie expenditure. Store your SexEx wardrobe in or near the bedroom to avoid any delays. Any additional devices that you will wear (ankle weights, make-up, heart monitor, ropes) or need (camera, pillows, video recorder, stool, metronome, vibrator[24], step-ladder, sphygmomanometer) should be close at hand. If you will be using the laughing techniques discussed in Chapter 6, cue up your records, CDs or tapes and set out your choice of funny pictures and posters. Any lubricants and perfumes, should be conveniently at hand. Place clean-up materials near by also. Only some of the foods and beverages that you will take before, during and after SexEx can be kept in the bedroom. Non-perishables, such as trail mix and bottled water, can be stored in a dresser. If there is a phone in the room, unplug it or silence it in some way.

Near to the "bedroom" there should be a bathroom with a shower or bathtub or at least a large sink. Even Vatsyayana many centuries ago recommended washing after coitus. This can help prevent infections and rashes as well as remove semen splotches (we all know how troublesome they can be) and sweat. You may want to cuddle or go to sleep, but proper hygiene is important, especially for women, to avoid irritations and urinary-tract infections (UTIs).[25]

The single most important piece of "equipment" is your birth-control device. You may keep some things in other rooms, but your birth control measures must be within arm's reach. In the throes of arousal, it may be OK to decide not to put on your ankle weights because you would have to go downstairs to get them, but it is NEVER OK to not use birth control unless you are deliberately trying to conceive.

Chapter 14

Swell-Wimp and Older People

Why is there a separate chapter for older people?[1] Can't or shouldn't they do what is described elsewhere in the book? Yes, they can, but age does bring with it certain limitations, even problems. Kinsey points out that "age is one biologic factor that most strongly affects variation in the sex life of an individual."[2] As you age, muscle tone decreases and supportive structures weaken (your body begins to sag). Further, you often become more sedentary and thus, gain weight. Interestingly, the overall risk of being moderately overweight apparently diminishes with age, so you should not become alarmed if you put on a few pounds. However, "moderate" can easily become "excessive." Since your weight naturally drifts upward as you age (no one yet knows exactly why this is), Swell-Wimp can help you keep a steady weight.

In the fourteenth century, Giovanni Boccaccio wrote:

> Those who go about talking of my age simply show that they do not
> know a leek may have a white head and a green tail. But jesting apart,
> I reply seriously that I do not see why I should be ashamed of delighting
> in these things [amorous kisses and pleasant embraces and delicious
> couplings] until the end of my life....[3]

We often overlook the obvious truth of what he says.[4] The desire and need for sexual relations begin in childhood and continue to death. Older persons should not be ashamed of their sexual desires. Although they have different metabolic rates, different sexual abilities, special restrictions (such as fragile bones, less lubrication, frequent urination, softer and less easily sustained erections), and decreased gymnastic abilities, they need exercise and sex—Swell-Wimp—as much as anyone else. Maybe more.

The population of the United States is aging. There are thirty million people over sixty (one out of seven) and five thousand more people turn sixty every day.[5] At the turn of the century the average life expectancy was 47, so fewer people lived to old age and fewer still were healthy enough for an active sex life. Today, life expectancy is about 71 years.[6] Thus, the subject of "elder sex" will become important to almost everyone sooner or later.

Often older people believe that physical limitations prevent them from engaging in SexAct. However, we're all temporarily or permanently handicapped[7] in some way, more or less, whatever our age: we wear glasses or are blind; we have a weak sense of direction, balance or smell; we have false teeth or a false eye. It is a matter of degrees. Some cannot walk without the aid of a cane or dog and others cannot get through the day without the aid of alcohol or tranquilizers. A paraplegic may run her own company while another person with no obvious physical limitations may not be able to hold on to a job. It can be said (almost without qualification) that some kind of sexual activity is possible for everyone, more or less, convenient or inconvenient, simple or complex.[8]

There is no inherent physiological reason why sexual activity should stop at any age. You don't have to be an 18-year-old athlete to be fit for SexAct.[9] Heslinga says that it "may be surmised that coitus places a strain on a man [and an active female partner] similar to the ascent of a single flight of stairs which are not too steep. If this degree of effort cannot be tolerated then coitus has to be abandoned or ways must be found of taking it at a quieter pace...."[10] You don't really have to be any fitter than this for Swell-Wimp, although if you can't climb a single flight of stairs without pausing for a rest then you are fit enough only for SexAct, but not Swell-Wimp. You MUST consult a qualified health-care professional before beginning Swell-Wimp. Gochros claims that the examination should include a stress EKG and Hellerstein's Sexercise Tolerance Test (developed by Drs. H. E. Hellerstein and E. H. Friedman) which involves wearing monitors during sexual activities at home (28).[11]

Even when menstruation stops, ovulation may continue, so birth control should be continued until a year after the last period. What is true for young people is true for older people; you should take precautions to prevent conception (unless you are deliberately trying to conceive)[12] and transmission of disease.

Attitudes

Not long ago accurate information about sexual matters was difficult to obtain and there was a lot of misinformation around. The procreative years of most older people occurred before effective birth-control devices were widely available, so SexAct was overshadowed by the fear of apron flowers.[13] Also, justified fears about venereal disease, for which there were few effective treatments, affected sexual relations. Further, society in general was more prudish about sexual matters. SexAct between grandparents was considered perverse and masturbation was forbidden for everyone, including the young and old who need it most.[14] Less than 80% of females born before 1900 has manipulated the male genitalia manually, while 95% of the younger generation has. Only 29% of the older generation has made oral contacts with male genitalia; 57% of the younger has.[15] Such constraints continue to influence older people and it may be hard for them to give themselves freely, even impulsively, to sexual expression.

People in institutions act as they are expected to act: prisoners, treated like prisoners, act like prisoners and mental patients act like mental patients. Place them in a different environment and they act differently.[16] Teachers know that most students will work to expectations. Older people shouldn't accept the rigid, stereotyped, desexualized image of what they should be.[17] If you believe that you should not do this or cannot do that, you will fulfill your own expectations.[18]

Societal attitudes affect both older men and women. Masculinity is often equated with virility and sexual performance. As men age, they may not be able to perform as well or as often and, thus, may be seen (even by themselves) as less masculine. Self-doubt affects their sexual performance and their performance affects their attitude. It's a vicious circle. Femininity is associated with beauty; because women lose the beauty of youth (as do men), they may believe they are no longer attractive and may not maintain their appearances, thus becoming even less attractive. Another vicious circle. These circles can be broken but you must do it: you must believe in yourself.

There are other attitudes that older people need to modify. You want special consideration because of your age (the assumption being that you are frail, poor, sick and vulnerable). But you rebel against paying taxes to support good schools and programs that benefit children, who (though they may be obnoxious) are often more vulnerable than you, and who, if properly educated, will be able to support you in the way that you have become accustomed. Social Security benefits are derived from taxes on those who are currently working, not from taxes you paid while you were working.

And other pension benefits are derived from current investments, not from interest on premiums that you paid. If current and future workers do not do well, you will not do well. If you continue to refuse to support programs that help the young, sooner or later, the young are going to turn on you.

Many of you want a double standard: you don't want to be discriminated AGAINST because of your age, but you want to be discriminated FOR when it suits you. You want to be eligible for Social Security benefits just because you reach a certain age, even if you are wealthy. You want your health care to be paid for by the government, but don't support universal health care coverage or even free health care for children. Why should you be charged less to ride public transportation or to purchase automobile and pet licenses? You willingly accept reduced prices at movie theaters, restaurants and drug and grocery stores. True, these are commercial promotions to obtain your patronage, but have you no pride? Long-term charity is bad for the soul.

Being old is difficult, but it can also be wonderful in many ways. As we have said, older people have to contend with negative stereotypes. If you don't stop demanding that you be treated as a privileged class, contending with stereotypes will be the least of your worries. We fear there is going to be a backlash against older people as a group, unless you change your attitudes.

So, do not accept the stereotypes. All older people aren't poor or sick and feeble or even retired. Many of you still work; most of you are healthy, competent, flexible, useful people.[19] You have many of the same troubles and joys as younger persons. Some of you are sexy and most of you want and need SexAct.

The Benefits of SexAct for Older People

Vigorous pelvic thrusting keeps the muscles and joints of the entire spine in good condition. Circulation and breathing are improved. The increase in heart rate and blood pressure during SexAct are good for the cardiovascular system. And despite the many jokes about randy politicians, the incidence of death during intercourse is estimated at less than 1% of sudden coronary deaths (in a major study the rate was less than 0.3%).[20]

Regular SexAct stimulates testosterone production which prevents and alleviates angina pectoris (chest pain of unknown cause). There is some evidence that regular SexAct is good for those suffering from rheumatoid arthritis, probably because of the cortisone produced by the adrenal gland and because of the physical activity involved. Much of the crippling by rheumatoid arthritis results from inactivity.[21] SexAct keeps you in shape for SexAct. Dr. Reed Moskowitz notes that "sex releases tension and turns off the adrenaline system." During sexual activity, the nervous system releases endorphins (natural analgesics) which "create a healing, relaxing situation for the whole system, giving it a chance to regenerate."[22] Prolonged abstention from sexual activity in old age leads to shrinking of the sexual organs,[23] but "...a pattern of regular sexual activity helps preserve sexual functioning" (Gochros, 23). So, *usus promptos facit*—use it or lose it.

Sexual desire and need vary among individuals of all ages. As Gochros points out "sexual disinterest is a matter of concern only if you find it personally troubling or if it causes problems in relating to others" (7). Although, there are no psychological reasons why sexual desire and need should diminish with age, you should not worry if sex is less important to you than it once was. However, you should not deny the sexual urges you do have (assuming they are "normal").

In fact, not engaging in SexAct (at any age) "...may prolong arousal, causing psychological frustration that will probably produce some adverse physical effects" (Gochros, 29). For example, the pain that an arthritic person may experience during intercourse may be less important than the stress that may occur if that person avoids sex in order to avoid the pain.[24]

"Orgasm is a natural analgesic," says Beverly Whipple. In her studies, she has found that climaxing significantly raised a woman's threshold for pain. There is speculation that this is due to endorphins (activated by orgasm) traveling to receptor sites throughout the body and producing a morphine-like effect.[25]

Most women cease to be able to have children sometime after fifty and most men can't father children after seventy, but the sexual organs don't wear out. Reuben notes that sex and eating are renewable pleasures; they are enjoyable again and again. No one would expect an older person to eat only mush. You can and should enjoy delicious meals every day. Similarly, you can look forward to and enjoy sex every day (or week or month). Eating and sex may be two of the few pleasures that some older people have left. Don't diminish your existence by refusing them. Resuming sexual activity or increasing the level of sexual activity will expand your life. Sex is good for your mental attitude.

Sex among older persons offers the opportunity to express passion, affection, and admiration. It maintains high morale and enthusiasm and it may add romance to your life.

General Problems

Regular and pleasurable sexual activity by older males and females is complicated by many factors. Children may deny their aging parents a sex life, making it difficult for them to find the necessary privacy or treating them condescendingly, as senile or as big children. All of this makes it difficult for older men or women to maintain their own dignity and pride and respect their partners.

Gochros notes that "the nursing-home resident who has sexual needs is truly a member of a forgotten and neglected population" (Gochros, 59). Five to ten percent of persons over 65 live in homes for the aged, nursing homes, and other institutions. Sexual relationships are very difficult for them; usually there is no privacy, even for married couples. We advise that you speak to the administrators and insist that your needs must be met. Request times and places for sexual activities; negotiate with them; demand as a last resort; but demand if necessary.

Medications can interfere with sexual activity. For example, beta-blockers, which are used to slow the heartbeat and reduce high blood pressure, can decrease libido in men and women. Diuretics can make it difficult for men to sustain an erection. You should ask your physician about side effects. Sometimes a modification of dosage or a switch to a different medicine can result in a significant change in ability to engage in SexEx.

Many older people have limited financial resources.[26] The activities usually associated with finding and keeping a sexual partner—dining, dancing, dressing well, and going to parties, movies, and bars—may be beyond their means. Gochros points out that sex is among the pleasures in life which are free, but this is not true. In addition to the usual expenses of "courting," older women and men may need hormone supplements, lubricants, and so on. Still his point is well taken. As we've said before, Swell-Wimp is much cheaper than most other forms of exercise and a real bargain for those who are "poor."

Grief, due to the loss of a spouse, friend, or family member can be disabling (especially for women who live longer). Contempt between partners may arise from intimacy due to retirement. In addition to problems which beset both older men and women, there are some which affect only one sex or the other.

Frequently, as we age our long-term memories remain intact, but it becomes increasingly difficult to remember recent events. The problems associated with establishing opposite-sex relationships is exacerbated when we can't remember our prospective sweetheart's name or whether he or she was the one we watched *On*

Golden Pond with.[27] Health-food stores sell several concoctions that claim to improve memory but there are no reliable studies to support the claims. Research does show that remaining mentally-active can help preserve memory. There are thousands of way to do this, depending upon your past life and current situation. You can continue to do some of the things you used to do (including working part-time) or find new substitutes for activities you can no longer engage in. We will have more to say about this later in the chapter.[28]

Problems: Males

Older men must contend with declining physiological powers. The erotic response at 75 is one-quarter of the mean rating for age 65.[29] At about age 40, the cells of the testicles, which secrete testosterone, begin to break down and are replaced with scar tissue, so the output of the hormone diminishes and this has a number of effects. The beard thins and the voice gets higher. Some men even develop breasts; their adrenal glands produce estrogen and their body's hormonal balance changes. It takes an older man longer to obtain an erection and it may not be as large or hard or last as long as in previous years.[30]

There is also a reduction in the volume of seminal fluid. Younger men produce 3–5 ml of semen (1 teaspoon) every 24 hours while men over 50 produce 2–3 ml. Despite this, older men can experience extreme orgasmic pleasure just as younger men.[31]

Although interest in sex may diminish, sexual activity often increases as a result of anxiety. Men try to prove to their partner(s) and themselves that they are still virile. A vicious circle sometimes begins in middle age; once a man begins to question his sexual capabilities, the odds are that he will experience difficulty getting or keeping an erection.[32] Almost every man at some time is impotent and about one third suffer chronic or repeated impotence.[33] Given society's attitudes about virility and manliness, this can be very troublesome, even humiliating, for some men.[34] Impotence[35] can take several forms: a man may be unable to achieve an erection or it may fade as soon as sexual activity begins;[36] he may be able to achieve an erection but ejaculate only after a long period of sexual activity (*ejaculatio retardata*)[37] or be able to sustain an erection (for hours) but be unable to ejaculate at all (anejaculation or *psychogenic aspermia*; and he may ejaculate immediately upon entering the woman (*ejaculatio praecox*).

Impotence may result from illness—heart disease, diabetes,[38] hypertension—and injury, but often it is psychological or emotional in origin: stress,[39] fear,[40] neurosis,[41] and psychosis. It has no obvious cause and disappears in a short time. It may be nothing more than temporary "performance anxiety" due to awareness of one's age, a new sexual partner, pre-coital bragging or unrealistic expectations. This type of "impotence" can afflict females as well as males.

It's difficult to determine how much the various changes that occur with age are due simply to aging and how much to disease processes. Although hormones seem to be the major cause in women (and thus there is a distinct female menopause),[42] much of penis-related changes may be related to nutritive, oxygen- and blood-supply deficiencies because of hardening of the arteries. (Heart disease, for example, is three times as great in men as in women in the 45–64 age group.[43]) Whatever the cause, the biggest factor correlating with impotence is age.

Problems related to the prostate gland are not the result of excessive sexual activity. In men twenty to forty, it can become inflamed and cause a feeling of fullness and pain in the perineum between the testicles and the anus. The inflammation can be caused by pounding of the perineum (motorcycle riders, cowboys, truck drivers) and by sexual stimulation without gratification (priests, sailors, lawyers and elderly males). After 40, 60% of men experience some enlargement of the prostate which can block the urethra. Surgery may be required if the blockage becomes serious. The only change after prostate surgery is that semen is no longer ejaculated through the penis but is pushed backward into the bladder (retrograde ejaculation). Normal sexual activity can continue. Further, "evidence suggests that an active sex life preserves healthy prostate functioning" (Gochros, 44).

Although many believe that an older man with a strong sex drive must be a pervert, the average age of men convicted of child molestation is 27 (Gochros, 1). Still, men must deal with the stereotype of the aging, leering lecher.

What Can A Man Do?

If you are having trouble achieving or maintaining an erection, there are number of things you can do.[44] Your partner should massage your penis.[45] She can even stuff it into her vagina and flex her vaginal muscles until it becomes erect.

Try new positions. The rear-entry, lying-on-your-sides position is the gentlest position and can be managed with little or no erection. During intercourse, the woman can hold the penile skin (and foreskin if you have it) forcibly back with her finger and thumb at the root of the penis and keep it stretched; this speeds up ejaculation. However, an understanding, sympathetic, caring sexual partner seems to be most important. So, relax, get plenty of rest and exercise, and stop worrying.

Impotence can be psychologically devastating (especially to a sexually insecure man), so it should not be ignored.[46] If you suffer from some sort of impotence, DON'T PANIC.[47] Assume it is temporary and follow the advice above. As a last resort you can try the expensive pharmaceutical Viagra. So, if your impotence persists, see a physician, psychologist or sex therapist.[48] Before you do though, be aware that obesity itself can cause impotence in men. Swell-Wimp can help you lose weight which will make you healthier and may improve your erection, which will improve your sex life, which will make SexEx more fun so you will do it more often and lose more weight, and so on. Once you take the first step, things fall into place and each action has a cumulative and beneficial effect.

Problems: Females

Older women have their own set of problems to deal with. First among these is heart disease. In 1991, two large studies (one done at Harvard and the other done by several medical centers in collaboration) showed that men with heart disease are roughly twice as likely as women to receive aggressive, potentially life-saving treatments. Further, since 1910, more women have died of heart disease than of any other cause, yet researchers "have systematically and almost completely excluded women from studies of all aspects of coronary heart disease."[49] In clinical trials conducted over the past 30 years to evaluate treatments for heart attack, fewer than 20% of the total 151,000 subjects were women. This is despite the fact that heart medications have different effects on women and thus, study results cannot automatically be extrapolated to women. And, until recently studies of the links between alcohol and heart disease were done only on men even though it has been known for a long time that women metabolize alcohol more slowly.

In males, a heart attack is usually signaled by a pain or pressure in the center of the chest, but women often experience the pain in adjacent or related areas. They also experience nausea, lightheadedness, or sweating without chest pain. Thus, heart attacks are often misdiagnosed in women. The risk factors that apply to men also apply to women: high blood pressure, smoking, high blood cholesterol and blood triglycerides, diabetes, obesity, and inactivity. Long-term use of oral contraceptives is also a risk factor.

Estrogen offers women some protection from heart disease, but estrogen levels drop after menopause. Yet, women over 65, when they have the greatest heart-disease risk, have been almost totally excluded from heart studies. "A lack of sexual satisfaction should be considered for further study as a possible risk factor for heart disease," says Alexander Lowen; in a study of 100 women treated for heart attacks, 65 reported feeling sexual dissatisfaction before hospitalization.[50]

During menopause, the blood supply to the ovaries, which produce estrogen, stops: they die and are replaced with scar tissue. We have all heard of the horrors of "the change of life," but 60% of women experience no remarkable physical or emotional symptoms (Gochros, 12).[51] Most of the changes can be traced to the decline of hormones following menopause rather than to aging itself.[52] Some women continue to produce sex steroids in smaller quantities after menopause because they are produced in the adrenal glands as well as the ovaries. However, "older women experience little deterioration in the physical *capacity* for sex as they age" (Gochros, 11).

The most common sexual problem for older women is the inability to achieve orgasm (Gochros, 91), and it is usually due to the same things that prevent young women from achieving orgasm: tiredness, emotional upset, boredom, physical ailments, drugs, and lack of adequate stimulation of the clitoris. Women in good health can have orgasms well into their eighties.

The term "frigidity," which refers to a lack of sexual desire and/or response, is usually applied to women.[53] True female "frigidity" is not as common as true impotence. What was once called "frigidity" is now known to be the result of males' lack of sensitivity to women's needs, faulty male technique[54] and the failure of women to educate and assert themselves. Since the appearance of Viagra, (male) "impotence" has been replaced by "erectile dysfunction; the pejorative term "frigidity" should be replaced by an equally neutral term: "orgasmic impairment."

The degree of ignorance (derived from folklore, the locker room, Freud and arrogance) about female sexual response, even among physicians, is hard to believe. For example, Frank Caprio, a well-meaning physician, in his book *The Sexually Adequate Female* (New York: The Citadel Press, 1953) says that frigidity "involves the inability to achieve a vaginal orgasm during coitus" (15). His view is typical of the time and that view is still held by too many health-care professionals today. Caprio acknowledges that "friction against the clitoris as a result of coital movements during intercourse helps a woman achieve her orgasm" (73) and that this "adds to the ecstasy of intercourse" (75), but "when women are unable to experience a vaginal orgasm (coital climax), but can get one if the husband stimulates the clitoris with his finger [then] [s]uch a condition requires psychiatric consultation" (77)! Further, if a woman "prefers clitoral stimulation to any other form of sexual activity, she can be regarded as suffering from frigidity and requires psychiatric assistance" (78). He admits that "frigidity" is "very often caused by sexual incompetence in the man" (15), but he means that a competent man should be able to bring his woman to climax during intercourse (the proper time) by delaying his own climax until she has received sufficient vaginal stimulation, not that he should understand that there is no difference between a clitoral and vaginal orgasm and that stimulation of the clitoris is the best thing he can do to help his partner reach climax.

Caprio acknowledges that women are capable of experiencing as much sexual desire as men and that some women can enjoy several orgasms in the course of a single sex act, but concludes that "this would tend to support the theory that frigid women are *blocked* from enjoying sex because of their inhibitions, repressions," etc. (83–84). Orgasm apparently has less to do with physical stimulation than "her attitude toward intercourse, her power of concentration, her willingness to cooperate, the extent of her wanting to enjoy sex relations and her ability to abandon herself completely to the pleasurable sensation of the sex act" (79).

He says that there is a kind of frigidity "common to women who are able to become sexually aroused by preliminary love-making, and who experience a sexual wetness [lushing] following stimulation but who cool off quickly once intercourse has begun" (90). It is obvious that he is describing a common situation in which the woman's arousal—by clitoral stimulation during foreplay—subsides once intercourse begins and clitoral stimulation is reduced. But Caprio says that "psychologically and emotionally these women are virgin-wives" (90) rather than normal women responding appropriately to reduced clitoral stimulation. What is the cure for frigidity according to Caprio? Psychoanalysis, of course, for serious cases. But first the woman should be a companion to her husband, take interest in his job or profession, encourage and inspire him, avoid complaining, and avoid competing with him. She can "maintain her individuality, a thinking brain of her own and still know how to advise her husband without his feeling that she wants to wear the pants. ...[M]en prefer a wife who is aggressive sexually after he has once initiated the advance" (41–43). That is, she should know her place and do all she can to get her husband to want to make her feel good so that he will delay his pleasure until she is stimulated enough to climax.

As foolish as all this sounds, you should remember that Caprio's discussion of the problem was enlightened for the time (although with a Freudian bias). He acknowledges that women can, want to, and should achieve orgasm. He places some of the blame on the male. And he admits that the causes of orgasmic impairment are complex and that it is curable (not a permanent personality trait or inherent element of femaleness). Unfortunately, too many people still believe the other nonsense he puts forward with medical certainty.[55]

Female orgasmic impairment as with male impotence can have organic causes (lesions of the pelvic organs, illness, and medications, for example) or emotional/psychological causes. Stress and tiredness can cause temporary impairment. It may result from a lack of knowledge on the part of the male partner or even the female. Long-term impairment may be the result of neurosis and psychosis as with male impotence and should it persist it requires medical attention.

As women age, the vagina may become drier as lubrication lessens. With the loss of estrogen, the diminished vaginal secretions become less acidic increasing the possibility of infection. The lining of the vagina thins which may cause pain, cracking and bleeding during intercourse. Because of the thinner vaginal walls, the bladder and urethra are less able to absorb the shock of a thrusting penis and may be irritated during intercourse, and the bladder may become inflamed by jostling.

The vaginal labia may become less firm and the covering of the clitoris and the fat pad in the hair-covered pubic area lose some fatty tissue leaving the clitoris less protected and more easily irritated. Changes in the clitoris occur.[56]

Female breasts are revered as sex objects but they shrink and sag as a woman ages and some women have had part or all of one or both breasts removed. This may affect a woman's (and her partner's) view of herself, but it results in no physiological changes in regards to SexAct. A hysterectomy[57] can result in pain if intercourse is resumed too soon; otherwise, it has no effect on any part of the vagina involved in intercourse.

Often, the worst effects of aging are not physical, but psychological. Women maintain their interest in sex longer than men. But

> [o]ne of the tragedies which appears in a number of the marriages
> [or any long-term sexual relationship] originates in the fact that
> the male may be most desirous of sexual contact in his early years,
> while the responses of the female are still undeveloped and while
> she is still struggling to free herself from the acquired inhibitions which
> prevent her from participating freely in the marital activity. But over the
> years most females become less inhibited and develop an interest in sexual
> relations which they may then maintain until they are in their fifties or even

sixties. But by then the responses of the average male may have dropped so considerably that his interest in coitus, and especially in coitus with a wife who has previously objected to the frequencies of his requests, may have sharply declined.[58]

The departure of the children from the home may cause depression and listlessness (the empty-nest syndrome).[59] And many women must face the end of their child-rearing years as single parents.[60]

What Can A Woman Do?

For women who have had a mastectomy, a properly fitting prosthetic bra can help relieve worries about appearance and compensate for the weight of the missing breast(s). Surgical implants can restore breast size and shape. Saline implants are safe, but the verdict is still out (we believe) concerning the long-term safety of silicon-gel implants which do a better job of mimicking the weight and consistency of the female breast. The FDA restricted their use after a number of studies indicated that they adversely affect the woman's health. Further studies (and meta-studies) have concluded that they are both safe and unsafe. So get the very latest information, consult a knowledgeable health-care professional and think long and hard before choosing silicone-gel implants. It should be noted that the loss of a breast in no way affects one's sexual desires, needs or abilities.[61]

Thinning of the vaginal walls, loss of vaginal elasticity, vaginitis and dryness all respond to local applications of estrogen creams and suppositories. Kegel exercises are useful for stress incontinence and strengthening the vaginal muscles in general.[62]

There is evidence that estrogen (via tablets or injection) can protect against heart attack, gout, hardening of the arteries, and osteoporosis. If progesterone is given with estrogen, some post-menopausal women resume menstruating. If testosterone is given with estrogen, hot flashes (caused by dilation of blood vessels at the skin's surface) can be eliminated and the texture of vaginal lining improved.[63]

Water-soluble lubricants reduce vaginal dryness and friction. You should not use petroleum jelly; it does not dissolve in water and can be a vehicle for vaginal infections (as well as destroying condoms).

There are several ways to reduce susceptibility to vaginal infections. Carefully wash the vaginal area and penis with soap and water before sex. Drinking large amounts of water and urinating frequently flush disease agents, and older women should micturate before sex since a full bladder is more easily irritated. Wearing cotton panties, no panties or heavier men's cotton shorts rather than nonabsorbent nylon or other synthetics can help prevent infections by allowing air to circulate in the vaginal area.

Some older women have never experienced orgasm because love-making was too quick and mechanical. If you and your partner still tend to have "quickies," slow down. Your partner must learn what pleases you. Use a lubricant if necessary; try new positions; take your time; carefully stimulate the clitoris. However, orgasmic impairment is usually a temporary condition and, as with male erectile dysfunction, an understanding, sympathetic, caring sexual partner seems to be the most important aspect of recovery. He or she should concentrate on doing those things which maximize your pleasure in a non-stressful manner. So, relax, get plenty of rest and exercise, and stop worrying.[64]

Tips for Older People

The first thing that both sexes should do is strengthen their backs. The back muscles are weaker in older persons due to general deterioration of muscle strength and the sedentary lives that many live. Further, after a lifetime of living, many older persons have chronic back problems (chronic strains, slipped or compressed disks, deterioration of the spinal column and so on). Thus, often the back is the body part that most interferes with pleasurable sexual activity. You should be sure to read the section on strengthening the back in Chapter 8 and you should avoid any positions that place an extra strain on the back. As Gochros say, "Sexual activity itself is an excellent form of exercise therapy for the back, stomach and pelvic muscles and if undertaken in a regular and reasonably vigorous manner can help reduce back pain" (33). And Teresa Brady, executive director of the Minneapolis Arthritis Institute, points out that the endorphins activated by orgasm "can soothe a multitude of hurts, anything from a toothache to back pain."[65]

The penis doesn't grow longer as you age to compensate for increasingly protruding abdomens. You may need to try positions that allow the penis to more easily reach the vagina, such as the rear-entry, lying-on-your-side position.[66] If only the male is obese, he can lie on his back while the woman sits astride his penis facing forward or backward. Or, he can lie face-up over the edge of the bed with his feet on the floor while the female stands astride his pelvic region.[67] The best thing you can do if obesity makes SexEx difficult is lose weight. So do the best you can, expend as many calories as possible, and SexEx will become easier and more pleasurable.

Depending upon your medical condition, you may have to find positions that accommodate wires, catheters, braces, clamps and so on. If imagination fails you, purchase an illustrated manual where you are sure to find a position that meets your needs.[68]

Except for a few changes, you should set up your bedroom as we advise in Chapter 13.[69] Even if you sleep apart because of illness or snoring, you still need a firm double bed for SexEx; a single bed is too restrictive (narrow) for SexEx by most older couples. Lining up your medications and denture container on the night table can put a real damper on sexual arousal. Keep any medications that you might need in a handy but unobtrusive location. It is a good idea to have a telephone handy for emergencies, but a phone can cause problems as we point out in Chapter 13. Pictures of family members can be disconcerting to a new lover.

You may have to carefully time your Swell-Wimp sessions—between medications, treatments and evacuations. This may result in less spontaneity, but that is often overrated. Remember that most people are restricted by the need to work, sleep, eat, and take care of children. They must plan their SexActs; few are able to spontaneously partake. In fact, most people fall into a routine—nooky on Tuesday and Thursday nights or Sunday afternoons, for example. Your need to find appropriate times and places is not unusual.

Extended Life Spans

There is considerable interest today in programs that claim to extend your life span. How long can people live? No one really knows. Bristlecone pine trees, sea anemones, rockfish and some shellfish do not deteriorate with age; only environmental disruptions and predators kill them. Thus, there seems to be no inherent reason for living things (plant or animal) to eventually die. Then why don't we live forever? Michael Rose of the University of California at Irvine suggests that evolution makes sure a living creature is around long enough to reproduce; anything unfavorable (like illness or death) that happens after reproduction is inconsequential. Things die because there is no reason for them to live after they procreate. Thus, we die, not because we must "wear out," but because the systems that prevent deterioration, illness and death before procreation cease to function as well or at all afterwards.[70]

Recently, significant research has been done in this area. In one study, elderly men were given injections of the human growth hormone, and, in general, they gained muscle mass, lost fat and felt stronger and fitter. But the effects disappeared when the injections stopped and there is no proof that the men would have lived longer if the injections had continued. Mice fed DHEA (a natural hormone whose level declines as we age apparently preventing the immune system from getting instruction needed to combat illness) were able to fend off cancerous tumors. Trials have begun with elderly people.[71]

Can Swell-Wimp help you to live longer? Of course. Any program that combines moderate exercise and a sensible diet can; you'll simply be less likely to die early of heart disease or cirrhosis of the liver, for example.[72] However, in controlled studies no longevity program has proven completely effective in extending the life spans of humans.[73] There have been experiments in which rodents were fed a very low-calorie diet—40% fewer calories than normal. They lived up to 50% longer than the oldest rats eating a typical laboratory diet.[74] In fact, "calorie restriction is the *only* method that has been repeatedly shown to increase the maximum life-span of mammals," says Richard Weindruch, of the University of Wisconsin.[75] Roy Walford claims that a low-calorie regime would also work for humans, and there are, in fact, people now conducting experiments on themselves: they are trying to live on a very low-calorie diet, hoping to extend their life spans. However, William R. Clark points out that it is probably not caloric restriction that extends life, but excessive caloric intake that shortens it.[76] Tom Kirkwood pretty much sums up what we really know about extending the human life span: we can live longer, healthier lives by: eating a lot of vegetables, fruit and fish; exercising and copulating (he doesn't mention Swell-Wimp); drinking a little red wine; and avoiding red meat, fatty foods and tobacco.[77]

Neither low-calorie diets nor Swell-Wimp has been proven to help humans live longer. Most people hope to live long, productive and interesting lives and regular exercise, which is at the core of Swell-Wimp, has been proven to improve the *quality* of life. So if you are going to experiment, why not try Swell-Wimp?

Further, Reubin Andres, clinical director of the National Institute on Aging, has determined that in middle age and beyond, people with higher weights have a survival advantage (based on Metropolitan Life Insurance Company "desirable weight tables" and other sources). He says that it's desirable to gain about a pound a year after age thirty, as most people do naturally. But it seems to us that an eighty-year-old person who is fifty pounds overweight cannot be said to be healthy. You can maximize your chances at longevity by following risk-reduction strategies: eat a well-balanced diet; exercise regularly; refrain from smoking and alcohol abuse; and avoid obesity.[78]

As is true of anyone engaging in Swell-Wimp, you should maintain a proper diet in order to stay healthy and energetic.[79] Many of the foods that older people eat to maintain regularity—prunes, bran, fruit juices—are excellent sources of energy.[80] See Chapter 12 for more information about diet.

Oral sex is pleasurable and avoids many of the problems associated with coitus.[81] It also expends calories. Fellatio can be substituted for coitus if there is a problem with achieving or maintaining an erection. The tongue is naturally lubricated and less likely to bruise the clitoris, so cunnilingus is an excellent way to bring an older woman to orgasm. Remember to wash the genitals and clean the mouth before engaging in oral sex.

Masters and Johnson report that a *Playboy* survey showed that 72% of young married husbands masturbated with an average frequency of 24 times per year and 68% of young wives were actively involved in masturbation averaging 10 times a year. A *Redbook* survey reported similar findings; even among older married couples masturbation continues as a common type of sexual behavior (296). If you (for whatever reason) have no sexual partner[82] or if your partner is not available (traveling or in the hospital),[83] masturbation can provide sexual outlet. There is no need to be concerned or ashamed, unless you do so frequently even though a sexual partner (especially your spouse) is readily available and willing.

Locating a partner can be the most frustrating aspect of sexual relations for older people. You can find one the same way other people do—through various social interactions. Get out as often as you can. Meet people. Remember that good-looking, sexy young people often make fools of themselves and are frequently turned down. Attitude is very important to the success of Swell-Wimp. Do not get in the habit of attributing every failure in your life to age. You might be turned down because he doesn't like your red hair or she doesn't like your mustache.

Still, it may be more difficult for older persons to attract partners, because they may have difficulty getting around (to meet people), they are less attractive, many of their friends and partners have died, and they often have less money.[84] However, you have lots of free time. And time is money. You can "buy" things with time just as you can with money. You have the time to take your time in developing relationships (sexual and otherwise). It may take you longer to do things, but you have the time to do things you couldn't when you were younger. Although you have free time each day, you have fewer days left. So don't waste them being depressed and angry. You have the time to find a partner (and value your partner) and the time to lose weight and tone up. You have the time to appreciate your new fitness and savor your sexual experiences.

Sexual attraction is for the most part physical:[85] you want to have sex with someone primarily because of the way he or she looks, not because he or she is smart or has a large pension. However, appearance is more than having big, firm breasts or bulging biceps. Older people, who are otherwise healthy, sometimes neglect basic, daily hygiene. You should bathe, shave, and maintain your hair, teeth, nails and skin. The amount of your sexual activity may be related to the availability of a willing and able partner, and appearance and hygiene are important factors to finding and keeping a partner.

It must be admitted that older people are just not as attractive as young people: their skin is not smooth and supple but dry and wrinkled; often their bellies and breasts sag and their upper arms sway when they move; they have liver spots, hairy ears and varicose veins; their hair is not thick and shiny;[86] they are usually less graceful; often their eyesight and hearing is weak. And they are not callipygous.[87] However, you must work with what you have. Since it may be difficult for you to find a partner, why make things even harder by shuffling about with your mouth hanging open? Men, more than women, seem to lose interest in their personal appearance as they age, but both sexes must be vigilant that they do not become "A tattered coat upon a stick" "Stumping upon a Cane."[88] You don't have to spend a lot of money on clothes,[89] but old boxer shorts and ragged nightgowns are sexual turn-offs.

DON'T DRESS LIKE THE YOUNG. You don't have to wear "old-lady dresses" or baggy trousers, but you shouldn't be wearing deliberately-ripped jeans or humongous, clunky sneakers. Likewise, you should not have your partner's name shaved onto your head. There is a time when people need to rebel and this expresses itself in the way they dress. It is a silly form of rebellion, but harmless, necessary and generally tolerable. As older, wiser citizens you do not need to rebel in this manner. You do not need (or generally want) to identify with rebellious teenagers (although you may want to identify with some of their causes). You do not need or want to assert your identity by looking silly.

You also do not want to wear the clothing that you wore in your youth (when you were rebelling or searching for your identity); it is probably inappropriate now (zoot suits, poodle skirts, a pack of cigarettes rolled in the sleeve of a T-shirt, sack dresses). There are companies that sell stylish clothing specially made for those who are confined to wheelchairs, those who wear braces, and those with other types of physical limitations. Older persons should dress cleanly and attractively with style, taste and dignity.[90] AVOID POLYESTER.

May-December Relationships

You shouldn't restrict yourself regarding the age of the partners you seek; don't worry if you prefer partners who are substantially younger or older than you—a May-December relationship.[91] The pool of potential same-age sexual partners shrinks as you grow older (due to death). Of course, older people also look for younger partners because they are usually more attractive and energetic. No one can definitely say that ten, seventeen or twenty-seven years difference between partners is too much. However, if you have to buy new school clothes each Fall for your partner, he or she is probably too young.

Since males are chronically less mature than women, younger women often seek chronologically older partners because they may be their maturational equals and can provide stability and security. But, older women may find it difficult to find sexual partners near their own age, because they live longer and because tradition holds that women should be younger than their partners.[92] In 1970 half of all women over 60 were widows while only 15% of men were (Gochros, 97). Further, an age difference of ten to twenty years between partners is still considered more acceptable if the man is older; thus, it is easier for a man to take on a much younger partner.[93] Still, older women, no longer needing the security an older man can offer, frequently seek the vitality and endurance of a younger man.

Often May-December relationships are built on symbiosis; each provides the other with something he or she needs. The younger partner offers physical youth and positive feedback; the older may provide a place to live, financial help, advice and wisdom. Frequently, both sexes seek younger partners because they find the opposite sex of their age unattractive.

Almost always, the younger partner is physically fitter. Both partners must take this into consideration. The younger must remember that the older may not be able to keep up physically. The older must not get "into an ego thing" and try to prove himself or herself physically equal. Gochros points out that "the longer you love, the more you learn" (240). What the older partner may lack in power, flexibility or endurance, he or she often makes up in experience and technique. May-December relationships are as well suited to Swell-Wimp as those between comparably-aged partners.

Conclusion

It should not be overlooked that there are some advantages to old age in regards to sex. Occupational stress is generally greatly reduced. Flowering aprons need no longer be feared. The problems and associated stresses of child rearing are gone. Further, many older people have lots of free time and thus can engage in sexual activity more frequently, for longer periods and when they wish. All in all things balance out. And, since "preliminary studies suggest that sex can bolster the immune system, relieve pain, ease some types of migraine headaches and have psychological benefits as well,"[94] it would be foolish to exclude sex. A full and satisfying sex life can be a normal part of an older person's life.

Chaucer's Wife of Bath asks "What thyng is it that wommen moost desiren" (l 905). She answers that "Wommen desiren to have sovereynetee/ As wel over hir housbond as hir love,/ Anf for to been in maistrie hym above" (ll. 1038–1040). Today the Wife of Bath might say that what a woman (of any age) wants most is a partner with whom she can regularly achieve orgasm. And this is what most males want too.

Chapter 15

Conclusion

And now for some *novissima verba*. Because of technical difficulties, we were unable to obtain consistent reliable measurements.[1] Lack of funding made it impossible for us to precisely determine how many calories are used during the various sexual activities describe in this book. We simply were unable to establish, for example, that wearing heavy clothing during coitus causes you to burn more calories than if you were nude. Published figures range from 80 calories per hour[2] to 480 calories per hour[3] for "normal" sexual activity. Throughout the book we have used the modest figure of 150 calories per hour[4]; using a higher number would have allowed us to make bolder claims for Swell-Wimp, but Swell-Wimp requires that you eat sensibly as well as exercise. If you take in 1,000 calories more than your normal activities require and you burn up 300 of them Swell-Wimping, you will still gain weight. Further, as we pointed out in Chapter 1, you must have a positive attitude and make a long-term committment. Swell-Wimp is not a "quickie" solution to obesity.

Common sense says that wearing more clothing, singing, adding weights to your body, increasing the room temperature and so on should result in increased caloric expenditure during SexAct. Indeed, it would be contrary to human physiology and the universal laws of physics if it were not so. But, you must take our advice *cum grano salis.*[5]

As the narrator of Chaucer's *Canterbury Tales* says, "[E]ek men shal nat maken ernest of game."[6] You don't want to become a Swell-Wimp fanatic any more than you want to become a jogging fanatic. You can lose pounds by doing more work—burning (rather than storing as fat) more of the calories that you take in. Swell-Wimp can help you do this. So get it on to take 'em off.

However, Swell-Wimp must be fun; you should look forward to the pleasures, not dread the work. Boccaccio expresses the correct attitude:

> I have no doubt that others will say that the things related [in this book] are too full of jests and jokes, and that it ill befits a grave and weighty man to write such things. ...I confess I am weighty, and have often weighed myself. But, speaking to those who have not weighed me, I must observe that I am not grave but so light that I float in water.[7]

Our findings challenge orthodox theories about weight loss and sexual activity. Several people who read this book in manuscript said they were surprised that we had the "guts" to publish our results. It is true that there have been many obstacles and getting the information to the public has been difficult. But it has been a "labor of love." A friend who said he found the manuscript "astounding," brought to our attention the following passage from Horace's *Ars Poetica*:

> Parturient montes, nascetur ridiculus mus ad captandum vulgus. Non margaritas ante porcos auetor ignotus currente calamo. Mundus vult decipi castigat ridendo ergo mores satis verborum. Valete quantum valere potest, non est tanti, otium cum dignitate mortui non mordent. Leslie, raram facit misturam cum sapientia forma redolet lucernam; semel insaniuimus omnes pero timeo hominem unius libri. La farce est ouée. Unius dementia dementes efficit multos valete; ac plaudite; acta est fabula.

This sums up the aims of this book and our hopes for you. It can be rendered more succinctly in English as:

> It requires many words to make even a small book, but they who write for the common man do not cast pearls before swine. With a swiftly moving pen, they undeceive the world. The book is finished. Let it stand for what it is worth. May what [we] have written bring freedom and dignity and leisure to the reader.

Swell-Wimp—it's easy; it's natural; and it's funny!

Appendix A
Description of the Study

Introduction

At first, the research was funded from discretionary monies available through Dr. Bathous' academic department. After Dr. Flanders became co-director of the study, we were able to obtain some access to a laboratory, conference room and computer. The computer proved to be inadequate and too quickly the funds were depleted.

An entrepreneur offered to invest a sizable sum in exchange for documenting our study on film. We were unable to come to agreement regarding distribution of the film and the deal fell through. In order to continue the study, we were forced to beg, borrow, and steal and then use our own savings.

Of course, others have had difficulty obtaining funding for research similar to ours. Around 1988, the National Institute of Child Health and Development (NICHD) awarded a contract to Edward Laumann, dean of the Division of Social Sciences at the University of Chicago. He planned to update the outmoded Kinsey report and amass the kind of information that would guide public health decisions. His proposal was of high quality and NICHD was set to launch the study, but in 1989 Senator Jesse Helms (Republican from North Carolina) and Congressman William Dannemeyer (Republican from California) intervened and the Office of Management and Budget and the House Appropriations Committee withdrew funding for the project.[1]

In October 1990, Laumann applied for a grant from NICHD to do a more limited adult sex study. His proposal got a high priority, but again he did not receive funding. In September 1991 Senator Helms had introduced an amendment to the NIH appropriations bill to remove money for sex surveys from the budget. (He wanted the same dollar amount transferred to that portion of the Adolescent Family Life Act devoted to encouraging premarital celibacy.)

Other researchers at the Carolina Population Center (at the University of North Carolina) had designed a longitudinal study of teenage sexuality of the sort called for by the National Research Council. They planned to study teens' sexual behavior, ranging from contraceptive use to homosexual activities. NICHD gave it a high-priority. In 1991 they received the first year's funding for a 5-year survey of 24,000 teenagers and their parents. But in July 1991, Helms and Dannemeyer successfully pressured Secretary of Health and Human Services Louis Sullivan to cancel the project.[2]

In the Reagan-Bush years, it was almost impossible to obtain funding from the government for any research even remotely touching on sex. (You are, of course, aware of the ban on research using fetal tissue.) During the Clinton years the situation has improved only slightly. Many of the epidemiological models of the spread of sexually-transmitted diseases are based on insufficient and outmoded information, but studies that would have yielded the information necessary for dealing with health problems, such as AIDS, venereal disease and teenage pregnancy, were halted or denied funding entirely.

The political climate has also affected sources of private funding. You probably know that the maker of RU-486 has decided not to market it in the United States,[3] but you may not be aware that it has been impossible for scientists in the United States to even do research with RU-486 which, in addition to being an abortifactant, holds promise as an effective treatment of several conditions. Even corporations and private universities have been reluctant to fund "sexual" research.

Thus, you will not be surprised to learn that we have had to hide the subject of our research and that we have had to finance the study ourselves. Unlike Kinsey, we have had no problems with the medical establishment or the police, nor have there been turf fights with other disciplines—primarily, because few people knew what we were doing. However, because of the reactionary political climate in the United States and because there are more guns in this country than gas stations and because abortion clinics have been bombed and burned (and a physician killed) and because homosexuals are regularly beaten because they are homosexual, we have feared for our safety. Despite all this, we believe that we have been able to do "good science," although we have had to limit the scope of our research.

Methodology

Every activity burns calories; it is work. If more energy is expended (when we work) than is taken in (when we eat), weight loss will occur. Sexual activity burns calories because it is work.[4] But, when we started our study, we had no idea how many calories. So, one of our first considerations was to develop a method or methods of measuring energy expenditure.

Kinsey writes that "erotic arousal is a material phenomenon which involves an extended series of physical, physiological, and psychological changes. Many of these could be subjected to precise instrumental measurement if objectivity among scientists and public respect for scientific research allowed such laboratory investigation."[5] We attempted to make such direct measurements.

We anticipated that we would have to monitor a number of activities involving small amounts of energy, such as the resistance imparted to a penis inserted into a wet or dry vagina, the compressive force of thighs and vaginal walls, the accelerative force of a thrusting penis, and the hydraulic forces associated with ejaculation.[6] At first we used ergs, dynes and joules[7] as units of measurement.[8]

Also, we found several interesting studies related to our subject that used these units of measure. For example, an NIH study reported that each goosebump a person forms requires .3 erg of energy.[9] And a CDC study found that fidgeting can burn 100 to 800 joules[10] a day.[11]

However, we realized that our results, conveyed in terms of ergs and dynes, would be of little use to the average citizen. So we decided to use the more common calorie.[12] It too is a precise unit of measurement, but is used frequently to convey nutritional information to the general public. Thus, most people have some idea what a calorie is, at least in relative terms. That is, everyone knows that ice cream "has more calories" than celery and, thus, ice cream is "more fattening."

Our decision to switch to calories delayed our research: we had to obtain some new equipment,[13] convert the data to the new unit of measure and review and revise our methodology.

Although our equipment was state of the art, we encountered difficulty in obtaining accurate measurements. It is easy to measure friction or acceleration in the physics lab, but difficult to do so in the "bedroom."[14] Some equipment did not lend itself to being easily attached to our study subjects.

For example, during one session we attached a measuring device to the buttocks of Mr. Norbert to measure accelerative and deaccelerative forces.[15] The device weighed only 6 ounces but had to be attached with a strap.[16] We had also inserted a very small electronic sensor into the vagina of Harriet to measure friction. Unfortunately, the motions of coitus dislodged the electronic sensor. It became clear that only by surgically attaching the sensor would we be able to obtain the specific readings we desired and we were unable to do this.[17] The wires leading from the sensor and the accelerometer attached to the male's buttocks interfered with intercourse. Neither the male or female was able to continue to climax, so even the measurements regarding accelerative forces were incomplete. Despite repeated attempts, we were never able to find a way to obtain these particular measurements.

In another instance, we had designed a device to measure the compressive forces exerted by the female within the vagina during coitus. Unfortunately, only after we had inserted it did we realize that it left insufficient room for the penis.

Another sensor, designed to measure the rate of blood flow in the penis, was designed to slip around the shaft of the penis. When the subject achieved an erection, we found that the sensor had not been designed to expand and that the subject was in considerable pain. We were unable to design an inexpensive expandable device; the average pre-tumescent[18] and post-tumescent human male penis (despite the popular notions about how "well-hung" men are) is quite small, short and flaccid.[19] We could not find a subject who was willing to have the sensor stapled, sewn or glued to his penis.[20]

Our university does not have a facility for designing and constructing devices and tools for the science department. And even if it did, our need to keep "a low profile" would have prevented us from using its services. In our next study we hope to make use of non-invasive, non-destructive measuring methods, such as X-Ray, NMR, PET, MRI, ultra-sound, and so on. Such methods are common in industry where they are used to look for flaws in materials such as steel and glass without destroying or harming the material. These machines are enormously expensive, though, and there does not seem to be a second-hand market for them yet. Association with a major research institution will probably be necessary, although to date none has responded to our proposals.

Finally, none of the subjects "took to" the sensors; in fact, all but one complained vociferously. Their reluctant cooperation may have skewed the readings we obtained.

We did find that the design of the "bedroom" (as we called our research setting) was of little concern. Our subjects had no more trouble achieving arousal in our simulated bedroom than they had in other settings. Slow arousers and climaxers (self-declared) were still slow and vice versa. Whether we simulated a complete bedroom with rugs, bed, dresser, alarm clock and so on or asked them to perform in a motel room or a corner of the office, made no difference.[21] Thus, when we use the term "bedroom," we are using it as a broad term to refer to any of the sites where our studies were conducted.

It is well known in the scientific world that the researcher affects that which he or she studies.[22] That is, there is no such thing as complete objectivity nor can a researcher remain completely outside the area of study. For example, if a sociologist joins a motorcycle gang in order to study it, what he or she is actually studying is a motorcycle gang with a researcher as a member. Or if you study microbes through a microscope, you are really studying microscopic life on a slide with artificial light illuminating it. Thus, scientists must take into account their involvement and take measures (sometimes extreme) to factor out their involvement.

Ultimately, we found it impossible to do this completely. We began our research as a double-blind study, but were unable to see anything through the observation window. Even a single blind caused too much interference. A large one-way window-mirror might have worked, but we were unable to install one.[23] Eventually, we observed our subjects engaging in SexActs through a simple glass window and sometimes, when circumstances required especially close scrutiny, we observed from within the "bedroom" itself. Thus, we must admit that what we were really observing was couples engaged in SexActs while being observed.

This does not significantly affect our findings because, for the most part, we were studying physiological rather than the social and psychological aspects of sex. Still, we cannot really state whether people use more or less energy (and thus potentially lose more or less weight) when engaging in SexAct in the privacy of their chosen location. Our educated guess is that they use more because they are less likely to be inhibited by the presence of observers.[24]

We believe that participants in Swell-Wimp should give considerable attention to setting (unless they are professionals).[25] Any activity is more pleasurable in a pleasant setting. True sexual excitement, which leads to substantial energy expenditure, depends on many factors. Whatever can be done to skew these factors positively (appropriate music, sexy attire, correct temperature, and so on) should be done. For example, having intercourse next to a garbage dumpster probably holds little appeal to anyone except rats. Thus, we believe, although our clinical experience does not support this belief, that considerable attention should be paid to decorating the "bedroom" (see Chapter 13)

A total of thirteen persons served as subjects in our study.[26] The initial group was composed of seven enthusiastic volunteers (three males, four females). One male and one female were significantly overweight (20+ pounds). One male was moderately overweight (10+ pounds), one female was slightly overweight (3–5 pounds), one male was grossly overweight (35+ pounds), and one female was slightly underweight (3–5 pounds). Four persons dropped out of the study after two weeks (two males, two females) and four professionals were hired (two males, two females) on a per session basis.[27] When two of the professionals became unavailable,[28] the authors took their places.[29]

We eventually settled on the procedure of weighing the subjects before and after each session.[30] In order to measure fitness, all subjects (except the authors) were given a stress test[31] when they entered the study and when they left.[32] Finally, extensive data was compiled for each subject concerning his or her diet and activities during the study period. Cross-matrix correlation was applied to the data and T-sum and Simkin's multiple-regression analysis was used to verify the results.

Oblique polynomial inversion confirmed that there was good correlation between the study results and the personal assessments of the subjects. That is, those subjects who said they felt fitter and/or leaner were. The single exception to this was the male author who lost nineteen pounds (he was significantly overweight at the start of the study), but reported that he felt "sluggish," "harried," "tired," "bloated," and "burned-out."

Another female subject who lost only 1.2 pounds over the course of the study reported that she felt "great," "sexy," and "a new person." Although her weight loss and personal response do correlate, the very positiveness of her response is probably due, not to the weight loss but to (1) increased sexual activity during the study and (2) increased attention given to her as a subject of the study.[33]

Despite our having to abandon precise measurement of the many actions involved in SexAct, we can make some statements (reinforced by observational and anecdotal evidence): dry versus wet intercourse would require more energy expenditure on the part of the male, but wet intercourse involves more energy expenditure on the part of the female (creating, secreting and replacing the fluids). Rapid thrusting uses more energy than slow. Obese people expend more energy during SexAct than skinny people (assuming the same positions, activities and so on). Being on top uses more energy. In fact, any additional weight that you carry or support (weights, clothing, backpack) increases energy expenditure. Too frequent SexAct decreases pleasure and increases soreness and tiredness. No subject gained weight during the study. All showed slight (1–3 pounds) to significant (19+ pounds) weight loss. Thus, it might be concluded that informed, controlled, increased SexAct can result in weight loss.

Shere Hite conducted her study by distributing 100,000 questionnaires of which only 3000+ were returned. As mentioned earlier, Kinsey used interviews, not direct measurement. In addition to taking measurements before, during and after sexual activity, we also questioned the study participants. We asked them questions such as: How hard was it? Did you feel like you did a lot of work? Was it harder this way than that way? Are you tired? More tired than before? The responses to these questions correlated well with our measurements of energy expenditure.[34] It's possible that our inability to gather precise, verifiable data and the involvement of ourselves as study subjects may have resulted in dubious data and doubtful conclusions. The correlation of weight loss and experimental sexual exercise was 0.563 with a confidence factor of 97% due primarily to the small size of the sample (both participants and sessions).[35] So we can't be absolutely sure of our recommendations. Kinsey points out that the validity of extending to generalization, conclusions derived from a study depends upon the size and make-up of the sample population and the observational, experimental and statistical methods used. However, common sense says that there is a causal relationship between sexual exercise, energy expenditure and body weight, assuming other factors (diet, other forms of exercise, and so on) are controlled.

Appendix B

The Unknown Side of Emily Dickinson

It may seem unusual to sprinkle quotations from nineteenth-century poetry in a book whose subject is essentially modern—weight loss and weight maintenance—but Emily Dickinson's battle with obesity can serve as an inspiration to all of us.[1]

Dickinson's life, until the age of thirty-one, was unremarkable, although by today's standards, a little restricted; Amherst, where she lived, and her family were Calvinist—strict, staid, and hard-working. After 1861, when the man she loved, Rev. Charles Wadsworth, rejected her and moved to San Francisco to become pastor of Calvary Church, several things happened. First, she began to write poetry at a furious rate (80 poems in 1861 but 366 poems in 1862!). Second, she gained a tremendous amount of weight (a common result of overeating in order to comfort one's self). Third, she began to withdraw from the everyday world around her.

After a time, the pain of rejection by Wadsworth diminished. She reassessed her situation and did not like what she saw:

> I felt my life with both my hands
> I turned my Being round and round
> And paused at every pound
> I judged my features—jarred my hair—
> I pushed my dimples by, and waited—
> I told my self, "Take Courage, Friend—
> That—was a former time—[2]

Through will power and sexual activity she lost weight; Dickinson found a method that was easy, natural and fun. She took on several lovers, and for seventeen years she explored the world of erotic love (unknown to her until she was thirty-one). Her last lover (in 1878 when she was forty-eight) was Judge Otis Lord. However, she remained reclusive and eventually she rarely left her home even to visit friends.

The first collection of Dickinson's poetry was published in 1890 and it was not until 1955 that a reliable and complete edition appeared (edited by Thomas H. Johnson). So it is not unusual (although still annoying) that critics have not had time to understand and reconcile Emily, the prim and proper "Belle of Amherst" with the erotic poet who could write: "Wild Nights—Wild Nights! / Were I with thee / Wild Nights should be / Our luxury!" (Poem 249).[3] Although she wrote in the second half of the nineteenth century, she is a very modern poet and person.

Dickinson's poetry is known for its unconventionality, its cleverness and its wit (among other great qualities). But until now some of the autobiographical aspects of it have been generally ignored. A careful reading reveals many details of her life, including her exploration of erotic love and her struggle with obesity.

It is difficult for us today to explain why Emily had no real boyfriends and remained a virgin until she was about thirty and then, after being rejected by the first man she really loved, became intensely interested in the physical side of male/female relations.[4] I do not pretend to be a psychologist, but certain causes seem obvious: her mother was weak and subservient and her father was stern and demanding (although fair), the kind of man who could write to his bride-to-be that they should "prepare for a life of rational happiness" not "for a "life of *pleasure*!"[5]

Her father read only "lonely and rigorous books" and her mother apparently read nothing. Although they were not warm and loving in the modern manner, there is no evidence that they abused Emily, despite what she says in Poem 613: "…when a little Girl/They put me in a Closet—/Because they liked me 'still'." Some commentators, such as Toby Nates, Zinna Nockers and Noel Godin Lentarteur, take this as evidence that they were abusive (at least psychologically), but the context of the poem makes it clear that this was punishment for Emily being overly rambunctious.

Emily's younger sister Lavinia was a "coquette from her cradle, very pretty, with a piercing wit and a rather bandit tongue" (Bianchi, 13). Emily's lifelong friend, Helen Hunt Jackson, was a "siren" and "coquette"[6] and "worldly where Emily was secluded" (Bianchi, 74). However, her older brother, Austin, was a model young man and his father's favorite child.

Her hometown was sedate; her parents were strict; her sister and best friend were coquettes; and her brother was "perfect." Is it any wonder that she was unsure of her identity? Her intellect and disposition drove her to reject the role of prim and proper daughter—to want to enter the larger, more interesting and challenging world of men. But, there was no guidance from her mother or father.[7] Simply put, she had many of the qualities associated at the time with men (forcefulness, stubbornness, intelligence, and curiosity), but the roles assigned to females at the time did not allow her to use and express them. In Poem 801 she says that it is an easy thing to be a man and express yourself, but it would have been wrong for her to try to do the same: "I could have done a Sin/ And been Myself that easy Thing/ An independent Man."

Thus, Emily confused male and female roles. This was not a confusion of sexual roles; she was not a lesbian and, although she says in Poem 518 "My Bride had slipped away," there is no evidence that she was bisexual.[8] As a child, Emily said that her Aunt Elizabeth was "the only male relative on the female side of my family," (meaning strong and forceful). For Dickinson, "male" and "female" were not determined by gender, but by personality and character traits.

After Wadsworth left her, she wrote "I used to [wonder]—when [I was] a Boy" (Poem 389).[9] Three years later in a poem about a snake (a phallic symbol referred to as a "shaft" and "Bone[er]" that "rides" and "likes a Boggy Acre" [dark moist places, vaginae]), she wrote again "Yet when a Boy, and Barefoot—" (Poem 986). Thus, she acknowledges that as a child she often felt like a male and wanted to have male genitalia (although she felt apprehension), even though she had been forced to assume the role of virginal daughter and at times embraced it.[10]

Her relationship with Wadsworth was conventional. She kept her "male qualities" under control and hid her interest in the sexual and erotic. In the poem "Wild Nights," (249) written before Wadsworth rejected her, she reveals her inner self through symbolism. In it she inverts the usual Freudian symbolism, referring to herself as the boat that sails on a male sea: "Ah, the Sea!/ Might I but moor—Tonight—In Thee." This is very important because she had not yet thrown off her false role and it was only symbolically that she could admit that she would rather be a man.

In 1863 (a year after Wadsworth left), in "My Life had stood—a Loaded Gun—"(754), she assumes the role of a gun, always a phallic symbol. She had come to understand that she could not be the virginal daughter nor could she assume Lavinia's role of flirt and coquette. Her personality did not allow her to be like her friend of later life, Maria Whitner, a worldly woman who wore a red silk petticoat, and who was a scientific thinker and openly agnostic.[11] And, of course, she could not assume the role of a man due to biology and her strict Calvinist upbringing.[12] The man in the poem uses her (the gun) to hunt "Doe" (female deer). At night she (the gun) protects him against enemies instead of sleeping with him: "I guard My Master's Head—/'Tis better than the Eider-Duck's/ Deep Pillow—to have shared—".

Emily had kept herself under control and had played the virginal daughter and she had been rejected by the man she loved. Is it any wonder that Emily invented a new role for herself? She withdrew more and more from society in which there was no real place for her and devoted more and more time to her poetry and private life, in which she could be herself.[13] Society and the literary world of the time would not accept from a woman (certainly not publish) the kind of poetry she wrote.

Thomas Wentworth Higginson, a preacher, abolitionist, writer and "friend," claimed that her poetry was unpublishable.[14] Her sister-in-law, Susan, and a friend, Samuel Bowles, editor of the Springfield *Republican*, published one of her poems, "A narrow Fellow in the Grass," (986) without her knowledge as a joke on "fubsy tubby Em." (They completely missed the significance of the poem.)

She took to wearing only white[15] after the breakup of her affair with Wadsworth to assert that she still played the role of virgin; as a gesture, it was an ironic "poke in the eye" of the hypocritical world (including her family) that would not accept her and her views.[16] However, she secretly took on several lovers and explored the erotic world of physical love. Apparently her first lover had an unusually small penis and only when she took a second lover did she become fully conscious of the delights of sexual intercourse.[17]

She was never entirely a person at peace, but she did make a place for herself (within the larger world) in which she defined the roles. She could write what she wanted, unlike published female poets who were restricted to insipid and sentimental themes. In her place and time, for a woman to express skepticism, to be a free-thinker was practically a felony.[18] Because she had made the decision not to seek publication, she could even write more honestly than male poets (remember the hassles that Walt Whitman encountered). At the same time, she could be a passionate lover because she had established and continued to play the role of eccentric old maid; no one suspected her of anything sinful. Her niece says that she "did not want them even to suspect about her" (Bianchi, 75).

It must have been a terribly difficult thing for her, not to find her place as most of us do, but to MAKE a place for herself. She admits in a poem in 1862 that "Narcotics cannot still the Tooth/ That nibbles at the soul—" (Poem 501). The "Tooth," of course, are the doubts that gnaw at her soul, that could consume her if not removed. There is no evidence that Emily actually obtained and used narcotic, but it would not have been unusual (think of E. A. Poe, S. T. Coleridge and other troubled poets). She frequently took sleeping potions because of her fear of death and uncertain place in the world.[19] Certainly, she did not become an addict, because, as she says, "Memories—of Palm—/ Cannot be stifled—with Narcotic—/ Nor suppressed—with Balm" (Poem 492).

Many critics find in her poetry the major theme of renunciation. It is true that she often writes about this, but not as much as generally stated. She renounced (and wrote about) the then-accepted "normal" life of a husband and children.[20] And she did renounce the daring lives of the skeptical writer, the free-thinking traveler, the abolitionist, and the suffragette. But she did not renounce family nor writing; she included them on her own terms into her life and affirmed them.[21] She did not renounce the erotic side of life either, but chose to keep it secret, since it was even more dangerous to be openly passionate than free-thinking or skeptical.[22] Thus, her poetry is as much affirmative as negative.

After some years Dickinson abandoned partnered sexual activity, probably because she could satisfy her orgasmic needs herself (experienced, sophisticated male lovers were scarce in her locale). Further, having brought her weight problem under control, she knew that she could keep it under control without needing any further help from men. For Dickinson was, if nothing else, a woman of tremendous self-control. Ultimately, though, we will probably never know why for the second time she brought about a major change in her life, this time abandoning her secret life of sexual adventure.

Because she chose to write about her secret, sexual life in her poetry, we have a unique record, unlike anything else in American literature. As was stated earlier, she really belongs to the modern period rather than the nineteenth century and her comments and insights are still fresh and valuable. We have included them throughout the book where appropriate.[23]

Appendix C

Ask the Doctors

Question: I need to lose weight and I like sex, but some of your suggestions seem pretty crazy, like singing while wearing a football helmet, ice skates and a red, plaid Woolrich coat? I'm fairly conservative and am not sure what to do?

Answer: Don't worry. A brown coat will work just as well.

Question: Wouldn't it be a good idea to have one sexual partner for pleasure and another for losing weight? That way, for example, two fat people could concentrate on wearing the right clothes and doing the appropriate exercises so they could lose as much weight as possible. And each could have different partners for fun sex.

Answer: We believe this is not a good idea. If you have sex with a fat person, he or she should be someone you want to have sex with. If you are going to turn SexAct into exercise only, you might as well jog or lift weights. And, of course, such an arrangement could result in two (or more) unpleasant relationships, further decreasing the pleasures of sex. The fundamental idea behind Swell-Wimp is that you can lose weight by doing something inexpensive, easy, natural and pleasurable in moderation. Except in rare cases, having two sexual partners for two different purposes won't be easy or inexpensive.

Question: My girlfriend has agreed to help me lose weight. She's really excited about Swell-Wimp. In fact, she may be too enthusiastic. Sometimes she wants to do Swell-Wimp in an inappropriate location. I don't want to hurt her feelings, but it's embarrassing. I'd appreciate any advice you can give me.

Answer: Never look a gift horse in the mouth. Many spouses and significant others refuse to have anything to do with Swell-Wimp (apparently misunderstanding

what the program is all about). Except for legal considerations, there are no inappropriate times or places.

Question: I'm 69. How long can I continue Swell-Wimp?

Answer: If you use common sense and accommodate the changes the human
body undergoes as you age, you can Swell-Wimp up to the moment you die (and what
a way to go!).

Question: I'm 14 and overweight. When can I start Swell-Wimp?

Answer: You must be at least as old as your state's minimum requirement for con-
sensual sexual relationships. The decision to begin engaging in sexual activity is a
serious one and should not be based on the fact that your friends say you're a little
plump. There are moral and religious considerations and you must face that facts that
you might contract (or spread) a disease or become pregnant (or cause someone to
become pregnant). Abstinence is the best way to prevent pregnancy and venereal
infection. There should be no connection between loss of virginity and Swell-Wimp.
Besides, Swell-Wimp is not for beginners; you lose weight by modifying an activity
you already take part in. Despite the fact that our research clearly reveals the benefits
of Swell-Wimp, we don't advocate that it be made part of high-school health or physical education classes.

Question: I'm kind of nerdish and I have never been much good at finding sexual partners. When will your book on autoerotic Swell-Wimp be published?

Answer: We discuss autoeroticism briefly here and there throughout the book.
You can adapt many of the exercises, positions and techniques to no-partner SexEx.
Our other advice, concerning diet, clothing, taking precautions, and so on, is useful
whatever your sexual orientation. When we obtain funding, we will be able to investigate this very important topic. Your purchase of this book helps.

Question: I am 32, female, gay, attractive and overweight. Most of your book
involves heterosexual SexEx. Are you going to write something for me?

Answer: See the answer to the previous question.

Question: I'm overweight and in prison. How can I practice Swell-Wimp?

Answer: Basically, you can't without risking injury or death. Unfortunately, our
studies of autoerotic Swell-Wimp have not even begun, so we can't tell you to buy
our book on that subject. See our advice in the previous question. If that doesn't
help, you will have to try jogging or some other form of exercise and dieting until
you are released.

Question: That's not much help. I'm a lifer!

Answer: We're sorry to hear that. You'll just have to be patient. In the meantime you could urge others to purchase this book so that we can begin further research as soon as possible.

Question: Can't warming up without clothing be psychologically harmful to those who are fat and ashamed of their bodies?

Answer: The answer to this lies in something we wrote earlier: the success of any weight-loss and maintenance program depends more upon your attitude than any special diet or exercises. You may be embarrassed by your pendulous breasts, sagging scrotum, pot-belly, broad hips, or protruding buttocks, but you should be ashamed only if you do nothing about them. Since you are doing something, Swell-Wimp, you should not be ashamed. As Walt Whitman says in "Song of Myself," "Undrape! You are not guilty to me, nor stale nor discarded." Further, as you continue Swell-Wimp you will be less embarrassed as you lose weight and achieve fitness. Of course, if your partner is really turned off by the sight of your body, you can warm up alone or in the dark.

Question: Isn't it possible that naked Swell-Wimp might be psychologically harmful to those who have lost a body part—a leg or breast, for example—and those who have scars from medical operations or injuries?

Answer: You have only one body and you should love it. Love your body as a parent loves a child. The child may not always please you, it may get into trouble and it may even embarrass you sometimes, but it is yours and it deserves your love. There is no reason to be ashamed of your body because it is incomplete or scarred, unless the injuries were self-inflicted. Even in such a case, your new attitude, shown by the fact that you are attempting to improve your body, balances the fact that you tried to injure yourself. Face reality; all bodies are less than perfect. Yours may even be disgusting. But it is yours. And if you love it and take care of it, it will serve you (and your partners) well. As Alexander Pope says in *The Second Satire of the Second Book of Horace Paraphrased*: "Goose-rump'd, Hawk-nos'd, Swan-footed, is my Dear?/ They's praise her *Elbow, Heel,* or *Tip o' th' Ear*" (122–123) and "Give me a willing Nymph! 'tis all I care,/ Extremely clean, and tolerably fair,/ Her Shape her own, whatever Shape she have" (161-163). In other words, we all have some attractive features and everyone can be sexy whatever his or her shape. However, if your partner is really turned off by the sight of your body, you can warm up alone or in the dark.

Question: It would be easier to learn how to do Swell-Wimp if we could watch someone demonstrating the techniques. Why don't you sell a video to accompany the book?

Answer: We did try to come to agreement with an entrepreneur to produce video-tapes for us, but that did not work out (see Appendix A). Our only source of income, except for our university salaries, is this book, so we hope that you purchased the copy you are reading and that you will tell others to buy it. In our soon-to-start lectures, we will use slides so the audiences can see how the exercises are done. Of course, we can't use film or videotape because some state laws deem the naked human body pornographic if it moves on stage, but not if it remains stationary. Maybe if this book does well, we will be able to produce a video.

Question: Why aren't there at least illustrations in your book? It is hard to visualize the exercises from the descriptions.

Answer: There are no pictures or illustrations in this book because of funding. We wanted to produce a pop-up book with figures that you could move by pulling the tabs, but the publisher said it would be too expensive. Maybe the second edition will have illustrations.

Question: I'm not familiar with many (actually most) of the musical works you recommend as appropriate for SexEx in Chapter 6. I don't like or listen to rock and roll. Could you suggest some other songs?

Answer: If you re-read Chapter 6, you'll see that the musical works we list span the gamut from rock and roll to classical, from show tunes to country and western. We've compiled a long list of other "music to Swell-Wimp by." We'd like to release a CD. But permissions have to be obtained (musicians are notoriously fastidious), funding must be found and a thousand other details have to be taken care of. We barely managed to get this book published. One thing at a time, please!

Question: In your discussion of fellatio you never mention a blow job which is my favorite. Why not?

Answer: What do you mean, it's your favorite? There is no such thing. See "The Tongue" in Chapter 8.

Question: Your book is pretty hard on men. Are you being fair?

Answer: Here is a quotation from a former Leader of the Free World, a wealthy, Yale graduate: "Well, on the manhood thing, I'll put mine up against his anytime" (George Bush). Now try to imagine the level at which poor and uneducated males operate. Let me give you another example: there is a school district in West Moreland County in Pennsylvania called Derry Area School District. Do you believe that if women had been sitting on the board when the district consolidated they would have chosen that name? Men have been in charge of most things (including sexual practices) in most places for most of human history and the world seems to be in a pretty dreadful condition. You don't have to be a rocket-scientist to figure out that men bear most of the responsibility for the current, dreary state of affairs, including the problems of obesity in many countries and starvation in others. In male-dominated Japan oral contraceptives were legalized only recently. What brought about the change? The introduction of Viagra! See also the previous question.

Question: "Bath house" sounds like a made-up name. Are your names fake?

Answer: Yes and no. You can't imagine how difficult it is to become and remain a university professor today. There are so many groups that question your political correctness, the appropriateness of your research, your personal deportment, and so on. Since the Supreme Court's basis for protecting freedom of speech is instrumental rather than constitutive (not an intrinsic moral right, but an instrument for achieving good), what is good and how good can be achieved may change from week to week. Thus, we cannot be sure that what we write today will not be grounds for dismissal tomorrow. Since we are not independently wealthy, we do not want to lose our current positions (this is true even of Dr. Flanders who is no longer associated with the Swell-Wimp project, but who will receive royalties). I believe in Swell-Wimp and want to do further research, but, as you know, I have not had much luck obtaining funding so far. It is not certain that we would lose our positions if our identities became known to the university trustees, but "Clarissa" and I have each chosen a *noms de plume* (or more properly, given the political climate, *nom de guerre*).

Bathous is not pronounced like nor does it mean "bath house." It is derived from the Greek and means something like "of the deep"; the English word "bathos" is derived from the same root. My mother (whose name I won't reveal) very much admired the poet Alexander Pope and hoped that I, too, would become a famous poet (that is not likely to happen). I decided to use the name of Pope's good friend, Perry Bathous, who supported Pope even in the worst days of another politically-correct time (Pope was a Catholic during an anti-Catholic period in English history).

Incidentally, Dr. Flanders would probably reveal her true identity if we should be nominated for a National Book Award or Pulitzer Prize.

Question: I would like to try Swell-Wimp, but you advise us to do so much at one time—yell, laugh, do push-ups, wear motorcycle boots, a back-pack, and a blood pressure cuff.

Answer: Well, as Boccaccio says in *The Decameron* "there is no one, save God alone, who can do everything well and perfectly." Do the best you can. The blood pressure cuff is not necessary unless you have a heart problem.

Question: David Reuben claims that for orgasm to occur the full force of the body's entire nervous energy must be concentrated on the sexual organs; he says that no one has an orgasm while playing the violin, sorting laundry, and so on. If I try to do all the things you advocate, will I be too distracted to climax?

Answer: Well, Reuben is only partially correct; it is only just before and during orgasm that your attention must be totally focused. You can achieve orgasm while answering the phone, watching television or a film, attending a department meeting, riding a Ferris wheel, taking depositions and doing other activities that do not require total concentration. You can do energy expending activities during Swell-Wimp until just before orgasm. Then you will be unable to worry about anything but climaxing.

Question: I really enjoyed your book. As I do when I read fiction, I tried to visualize the characters acting and speaking. Why aren't there pictures of Dr. Bathous and Dr. Flanders on the back cover? They would have helped.

Answer: One of the articles of the agreement (28.d.3) arrived at between Dr. Flanders and myself when she disassociated herself from the Swell-Wimp Project, was that her identity would be protected (see the previous question about our *noms de plume*). She felt that posing for a picture "wearing a damn silly disguise" would "fool no one" and that it would be "demeaning." I tried reasoning with her, but she remained adamant. Although I had my picture ready to send to the publisher (and a damn *clever* disguise, it was), a broad interpretation of article 16.a.4 prohibited me from sending it.

Question: Some of your advice seem weird—even stupid. Do you really expect me to do this stuff?

Answer: Well, there are a lot of "stupider" things you could do, such as building your home in a flood plain, having a diamond embedded in your front tooth and reading Danielle Steele's books. And many of these dumb things cost a lot of money (paying $92,000 to get your picture taken with the President, smoking cigarettes, and dressing cool). We believe that Swell-Wimp is not a stupid thing to do. It will help you to lose weight and become fit. Anyway, as the ancients said *dulce est desipere in* *loco* (it is pleasant to act foolishly from time to time). Swell-Wimp doesn't cost much (just the price of this book). And it requires no more effort than other diet and/or exercise programs. So, since we all do "stupid" things, why not try Swell-Wimp?

Question: First, let me say that I am a Swell-Wimper; it's a wonderful program and it works! However, I almost didn't try it because I was put off by the disparaging remarks about members of Congress, doctors (excuse me, physicians) and lawyers in your book. It seems to me that these strident attacks serve no real purpose and might cause some people in need of Swell-Wimp (as I was) to not finish reading the book. Further, "putting down" those from whom you seek funding seems counter-productive.

Answer: I'm not sure what your question is, but let me quote Alexandar Pope. In *Epilogue to the Satires: Dialogue II* he writes: "As Hog to Hog in Huts of *Westphaly* [Washington D. C.];/ If one, thro' Nature's Bounty or his Lord's,/ Has what the frugal, dirty soil affords,/ From him the next receives it, thick or thin,/ As pure a Mess almost as it came in;/ The blessed Benefit, not there confin'd/ Drops to the third who nuzzles close behind;/ From tail to mouth, they feed and they carouse;/ The last full fairly gives it to the *House*." And in *The Second Satire of Dr. John Done* he writes: "Time, that at last matures a Clap to Pox,/ Whose gentle progress makes a Calf an Ox,/ And brings all natural events to pass,/ Hath made him an Attorney of an Ass." Do you know the percentage of lawyers in Congress?

Question: The mean age of first orgasm resulting in ejaculation is 13.88 years. By 15, 92% of males have had orgasm, but less than 25% of females. Further, the female population is 29 before it includes as high a percentage of experienced individuals as found in the male curve at 15. (This lag is apparently culturally caused, not due to physiological reasons.) Thus, it can be seen that males begin having sexual experiences at an earlier age than females and that they have more experiences. It seems to me that if left alone, women wouldn't become sexually active at an early age. But society values the wrong things—qualities that young men embody: strength, loyalty, aggressiveness, confidence and so on. Young girls are "hit on" by young males who represent society's best, the things it values. So they give in. This may demonstrate a weakness in women but it is an understandable weakness. Just look at former President Bush who thought that being a man meant acting like an 18-year-old male. Note his sports and fitness mania; his strong loyalty to inept, unethical and incompetent friends, colleagues and running mates; his smart-alecky use of language ("Read my lips," "Kicked ass," "Ozone Man," "Baghdad Bully"); his obvious joy at playing war; his simplistic, black-and-white view of the world (abortion: bad, bad; babies:

good; no new taxes: good; budget compromise: a mistake; Russia: former enemies, now friends; immigration of the poor to America: used to be good); and his lack of historical perspective. Does this sound like a world statesman or a male, high-school senior? And then there's President Clinton and Monica Lewinsky. Is it any wonder that young females give in to male pressure? Doesn't it seems clear that society's problems with rampant venereal disease and teenage pregnancy are caused by males—that girls receive an unfair portion of the blame, probably because pregnancy is so obviously visible?

Answer: Yes.

Question: How can I tell when my wife has an orgasm?

Answer: Hite claims that the female orgasm can be verified by the erection of the nipples afterwards, but this can also happen if the woman is simply aroused or cold. Late in the excitement phase or early in the plateau phase, a reddish, spotty skin color resembling measles develops in 50% to 75% of women and 25% of men, starting below the breast bone and spreading over the breasts and front of the chest and also the neck, buttocks, back, arms, legs and face. But this doesn't help in determining if the other 25% to 50% of women have had an orgasm. Since the clitoris often becomes very sensitive after orgasm, if your partner crosses her legs and tells you to get off, it may indicate that she has had an orgasm (or you have been engaging in clumsy foreplay for too long). There is really no way to absolutely determine whether a woman has achieved climax (the orgasm may be mild or she may fake it). Of course, you could ask her.

Question: Why was note 31 of Chapter 8 deleted? Who deleted it?

Answer: Answer deleted. [ed.]

Question: There is no question of the value of the male orgasm. Because it feels good, males want to do it a lot and thus pass on their genes frequently. Also, males probably achieve orgasm so quickly because their ancestors could avoid danger and devote more time to eating. But why is there a female orgasm? Why should women have the capacity for climax when they can make babies without it; what is the Darwinian adaptive value of the female orgasm?

Answer: This is a bit out of our field of expertise, but we will try to answer your question. There is no evidence that orgasm contributes to fertility or fecundity. It is known that orgasmic contractions do not suck the sperm into the uterus (as was once thought); in fact, they expel them. Even though it may feel good, repeated copulation does not increase the chances of a female passing on her genes. And the more time spent copulating, the less time that is available for eating and caring for off-spring. Some theorists speculate that orgasm keeps the female in position to ensure insemination, but this assumes that orgasm usually accompanies intercourse (which it does not).

It has been argued that orgasm helps the female establish a relationship with a net-work of males (rather than a single, best male), which helps prevent attacks upon her offspring. Females can experience more prolonged arousal and achieve orgasm more frequently than males. Because of the pleasure of the orgasm, a female will be promiscuous and mate with many males. If she doesn't climax with one, she will move on to another.

Others maintain that the female orgasm is an accident, a by-product like male nip-ples. It exists merely because the same trait in the opposite sex has some selective advantage; since the penis is so good for males, the clitoris, which develops from the same fetal tissue, cannot help but result in female orgasm. It may have no evolution-ary value; its only value may be pleasure. Female humans are always capable of sex-ual arousal and orgasm. Unlike males, they do not need orgasm in order to procreate. Thus, the pleasurable and utilitarian are separated. Orgasm may be nature's way of compensating women for the burdens of pregnancy, birth and child rearing. Or it may be proof that women have evolved beyond men and risen above necessity. No one knows. And one might ask, who cares? Women can achieve orgasm—repeatedly and frequently—without the participation of males. In other words a woman without a man is like a fish without a bicycle. Maybe the question should not be, why is there a female orgasm, but why is the male orgasm accompanied by ejaculation?

Question: Is there a Swell-Wimp Web site where I might get additional informa-tion? Do you have email addresses that I might send questions to?

Answer: We would like to set up a Web site, but we cannot afford to do so. As you may be aware, the Swell-Wimp Project is running on a shoe-string budget. No one in the Project knows enough about the Web to construct a site and we cannot afford to hire someone to do it. Our publisher says that they will "put up" some sort of site or page or something related to the book if it sells well enough (you did buy the copy you're reading, didn't you?). So check our publisher's Web site occasional-ly. The answer to the second part of your question is no. Do you realize how much email we would get if our addresses were public? Every dissatisfied reader would send us his or her complaint. Thousands of suggestions for the next edition and for other similar books would pour in. Every day there would be hundreds of questions from readers about things covered and not covered in the book. And we'd get who-knows-how-many messages from weird people who want to tell us about their sex lives. Would you want to read that stuff? Most people will not take the time to write a single letter but they will dash off dozens of badly-written email messages. Since Dr. Flanders is no longer associated with the Swell-Wimp Project, I would have to handle all the email myself. And I wouldn't earn a single additional penny even if I spent hours on-line every day. If you have a **serious** comment, question or suggestion, send it to me through my publisher.

Question: I recently visited a Web site called "Debbie Does Swell-Wimp" and enjoyed it very much. Was Debbie part of the original study or is she a new member of the Swell-Wimp Project?

Answer: No Debbie was or is associated with the Project. Further, there is NO official Swell-Wimp Web site nor has the Project officially associated itself with any Web site. "Swell-Wimp," and "SexEx" are in the process of being trademarked, so the operators of unauthorized sites will soon face legal action. We urge you not to patronize unauthorized sites such as "Illustrated Swell-Wimp," "Swell-Wimp: Get It On And On And On...," "Swell-Wimp SexEx-ercise," "Bathous and Flanders *au naturel*," "The Swell-Wimp Catalog Store," "The Swell Pimp," "Fashion Tips for Swell-Wimpers," and "Swell-Wimp for the Fetishist."

Question: In Chapter 1 you cite an article in a 1993 issue of *Consumer Reports* indicating that "yo-yo dieting" is harmful, but the January 1998 issue says, "While 'yo-yo dieting,' periodically losing and regaining weight, is no longer considered harmful to your health, it's obviously better to keep your weight permanently under control." How can we trust your information when some of it is clearly out-of-date?

Answer: First, if you check Chapter 1 again you will see that there is a note referring the reader to this question; thus, we do give the reader the very latest information. Second, trust? Trust whom? Look at the second part of the sentence you quote: "it's obviously better to keep your weight permanently under control." Obviously? Why do they say "obviously"? Physical scientists have learned not to assume that anything is obvious (the world is obviously flat, the sun obviously revolves around the earth, DDT and Thalidimide are obviously harmless, the atom is obviously indivisible, and so on) and in the social sciences, much of what was obvious (blacks and women are inferior, for example), was obviously wrong. You have to be watchful for junk science and junk-science reporting (although we like and respect *Consumer Reports*). Imagine the following scenario: a man weighs 155 pounds. During the eight or nine winter months he consumes a lot of beer and junk food while watching football and basketball on TV and generally enjoys life without giving any thought to his diet. Further he does no conscious exercising (no treadmill in his bedroom). The result: his weight goes up to 180 pounds. During the 3 or 4 summer months, he works outside gardening, cutting wood for the winter, repairing his house, and mowing his lawn, and he engages in a several play activities like swimming, playing softball and fishing. Further he eats lighter meals and lots of fresh fruits and vegetables as they come into season. The result: his weight comes down to 155 pounds again. Since yo-yo-ing isn't harmful, he has the best of both worlds: he eats what he wants and exercises when he wants and his weight never goes above 180 or below 150. Is this bad for him? *Consumer Reports* seems to say no, so why is it "obvious" that he should keep his weight permanently under control? Isn't this man's lifestyle in accord with the natural cycle for humans (the reverse of wild animals, who beef up in the summer and slim down in the winter)? Further, as we indicate in Chapter 14, Reubin Andres concludes that it's desirable to gain about a pound a year after age thirty, as most people do naturally. So why should this man try to keep his weight permanently at some arbitrary point in opposition to his genetic programming? We don't disagree that it's important to be aware of your weight and to keep it under control in general, which might include some yo-yo-ing. You must be on the look-out for sloppy science reporting like the sentence quoted above. Obvious? No scientist or science-writer should ever use that word. Further, notice that Swell-Wimp is not mentioned in the article on dieting books in the same issue. So, maybe the information in the January 1998 issue of *Consumer Reports* wasn't included because it's bad science or because it's biased. In any case, if it is true (although not obvious) that keeping "your weight permanently under control" is a good thing, then Swell-Wimp is the best "program" to help you do so. It's easy, it's natural and it's fun.

Question: I'm an enthusiastic Swell-Wimper and proud of it. Some of my friends are involved in things like Weight Watchers, Kiwanis, PTA, and so on and they let everybody know it by wearing caps and sweaters with logos and mottos on them. Where can I get a Swell-Wimp bumper sticker and baseball cap?

Answer: You can't, yet. We had hoped to make available a Swell-Wimp calendar (for record keeping), but hadn't given any thought to sweatshirts, coffee mugs, baseball caps and bumper stickers. Sounds like a good idea. Anyone interested in producing such items (nothing in bad taste, please), contact us through our publisher.

Question: It's really hard to find things in your book. For example, I know I read something about President Pierce, but I can't find it. Why don't you have an index?

Answer: Good indexing is very expensive. Electronic indexing (simply listing the pages on which a select group of words appear) is almost useless. Maybe the next edition will have an index. In the meantime do what all good students do. As you read underline significant words and phrases. Highlight interesting passages. Bend the corners of important pages. Make notes in the margins. Use sticky-notes as bookmarks. Are you sure there's a reference to President Pierce?

Notes

First Preface

1. Leslie La Bomba and I were attending Merry Forest College at that time and working closely on several projects, although I don't recall the particular circumstances that occasioned the remark. Leslie is currently the Vice Editor of *Steatopygia: The Journal of Advanced Propaedeutics*.

2. For example, Harley Warwick Lane, "Sexual Activity and the Middle-Aged By-Pass Patient," *The Journal of Near, Far and North-by-North Eastern Yonic Studies*, 10:78–94; Shelton Jackson Lee, "Mo" Better Sex," *People*, 13 June 1985, 23; Daniel Lamber, "Ergs and Nooky," *The Athletic Director* (The Hague: Poep & Stront, 1967), 121–34; Stephen Glass, "Sex Makes Me Sweat," *Hetaera*, April 1983, 51–52; Lynn Gahm Nayika, "Sweating," *Encyclopedia Sexualis* (Piltdown: Scitan Books, 1979), 34–35. William Denny, *Recreational Aspects of Sex and Mental Prophylaxis: A True Guide to Happiness* (Bremerhaven: Porter Books, 1931). Further, not a single work in Kinsey's extensive bibliographies addresses this topic.

3. See, for example, *The Homemaker's Calorie Chart*, United States Department of Health, Education and Welfare (GPO: 1968); Eman Ekaf, "Fattening Foods To Avoid During The Holiday," *Redbook*, December 1981, 67; Polly Himnia, "Build Your Own Ergometer," *Popular Mechanics*, June 1983, 67–73.

4. Dr. V. Atsya Yana, author of *Geriatric Weight Lifting* (New York: Bumfodden, 1979) and "A Caber a Day Keeps the Doctor Away," *Sports Medicine*, 12:321–44.

5. I was an Adjunct Professor at Our Lady of Cunegund College and awaiting notification regarding a NEA grant.

6. For reasons that I cannot make clear now, these are not their real names; however, they know who they are and to them I say "Thanks!"

Second Preface

1. *Scientific American*, January 1998, 34 & 60; *Discover*, January 1998, 104; *Consumer Reports*, January 1988, 22.

Third Preface

1. Vidal, *Myron* (NY: Random House, 1974); Boccaccio, *The Decameron*, trans. Richard Aldington (NY: Dell Publishing, 1930), 637.

Acknowledgments

1. We were saddened to learn that they had divorced after so many years.

2. We were surprised to learn from *Alfred C. Kinsey: a Public/Private Life* (W. W. Norton & Co., 1997) that Kinsey engaged in voyeurism, masochism (he circumcising himself without benefit of anesthesia), and other non-traditional sexual practices. The author, James H. Jones, adds "prurient needs" to Kinsey's motives for studying human sexuality, but concludes that Kinsey was a trailblazer who convinced us that human sexual behavior could and should be studied scientifically. We believe that researchers' personal motives and values must always be distinguished from their methods and data. As you will learn from the many citations in this book, good people can do bad science and bad people can do good science.

3. Even a great writer like Homer sometimes made mistakes. [ed.]

Introduction

1. Not "something extraordinary, new and never hit upon before," but "not new things but in a new way." [ed.]

2. You must take into account local laws concerning sexual activity. Almost everywhere prostitution is illegal, but only some locations have laws against oral sex. For example, you may live in such a backwater and the law may be enforced. Therefore, Swell-Wimp is void where prohibited.

3. In fact, it seems that it is the only study of its kind, but limited funding has prevented us from doing a comprehensive search of the literature (see Appendix A). Thus, there may be other similar studies, but if so, they must be very narrow and buried in obscure journals, since we have been unable to find them.

4. 15 November 1991.

5. 8 November 1991.

6. March 1992, Wilkes College, Wilkes-Barre, PA.

7. Critics, as William Empson points out in *Seven Types of Ambiguity*, are often "barking dogs...who merely relieve themselves against the flower of beauty..." (NY: Noonday Press, 1955, 12).

8. See Chapter 10, note 33.

Chapter 1

1. To holy places through narrow places; success after difficulties. "A fit motto for dieters" says Eugene Ehrlich, in *Amo, Amas, Amat and More* (NY: Harper and Row, 1985), 20.

2. *The New Joy of Sex* (NY: Crown Publishers, 1991), 79.

3. Did you know that the word "tabloid," often applied to sensationalist magazines (tabloid journalism), once referred to drugs taken in tablet form? And that "magazine" is derived from the Arabic for "storehouse"? And speaking of tabloids, a recent issue of *The Midnight Tatler* contained a story entitled "Cher's Agony as Owl Snatches Beloved Tabby." Agony? Really? Who cares enough to read such a story (true or not)? Who is paid enough to write such a story (true or not)? For an on-going analysis of mainstream journalism, see www.dailyhowler.com.

4. *The Midnight Tatler*, 16 March 1994; *Household Words*, 1 January 1991; *Ladies' Companion*, 8 August 1994. For an extreme example of a specialized diet, see Fulvio Tomizza's *Heavenly Supper: The Story of Maria Janis* (University of Chicago Press, 1991). Maria claimed to have survived for five years on a daily diet of communion wafers and wine. We've just come across a book by Margaret Danbrot called *The New Cabbage Soup Diet* (St. Martin's, 1997). My grandmother would be surprised to learn that cabbage can be the major ingredient in a weight-loss diet; she always said that it "put meat on your bones."

5. As we said earlier, we must speak plainly and avoid euphemisms (plump, stocky, overweight, heavy, corpulent, chubby, stout, portly, pudgy, obese). There are, of course, degrees of fatness, but we all know a fat person when we see one.

6. Studies have shown that repeated weight loss and gain are more harmful than simply remaining moderately overweight. An excellent article that summarizes the current state of knowledge concerning dieting is "Losing Weight: What Works. What Doesn't" in *Consumer Reports*, June 1993, 347–352. See also note 6.

7. Be sure to read Appendix C for the latest information on "yo-yo" dieting.

8 See the works of Frederick Madden and Norman Cohn concerning the extravagant claims made by some hustlers and the writings of Patricia Smith, Mike Barnicle and Vigdis Finnobogadottir for examples of attempts to "pull the wool" over readers' eyes.

9. See, for example, Cide H. Benengeli, "The Impossible Dream", *Beadle's Monthly* March 1977, 54–59 and John Ray, Jr., "She Couldn't Stay Small," *Cornell Studies*, 54:112–9.

10. There are, of course, thousands of factors, most of which cannot be quantified. For example, if the dieter dies before achieving his or her goal, should that be considered failure or success? Suppose an exerciser accidentally locks himself (or herself) in the basement. Then imagine that when he or she is rescued four days later he or she has lost 11 pounds. How does one categorize this weight loss? And there are so many other factors (removal of an organ during surgery, growing a beard, etc.)

11. Incidentally, Swell-Wimp is totally unrelated to Booberobics, which is not a system of exercises for increasing breast size, but a program for the clumsy and uncoordinated run by the Order of the Mammarites.

12. There are those who would object, saying that jogging can become a normal part of everyday life and that you can, in fact, jog no matter how old you are, but this is not true. Sooner or later, as you age you will discover that jogging is no longer possible, whether because your failing eyesight or hearing no longer allows you to run through city streets or because the rules do not allow you to leave the institution alone. See Chapter 14.

13. Juliet B. Schor, *The Overworked American: The Unexpected Decline of Leisure* (NY: Basic Books, 1992).

14. However, some forms of exercise may be, at least, partially tax-deductible. Golfing can combine exercise (sort of) with furthering your business interests and that portion devoted to entertaining clients is deductible. Thus, golf is very popular with lawyers. Except for some medical costs (examinations and VD treatments), sexual activity is not tax deductible. C. F.

15. Thus, you can worship the Lord and your body at the same time, I guess.

16. Sandra Fisher, a "wellness consultant," sells a cassette-based program called *Workout While U Drive* and Cyndi Targosz has a fitness cassette, *Drive to Fitness*, "created to use while you're driving [in an automobile]." These programs stretch the concept of "workout" to the limit. We believe that driving is a difficult and dangerous activity that requires your full attention; you shouldn't be trying to learn a new language, talking on the phone or "working out" (especially Swell-Wimping). Some self-help books address a very narrow audience: Dr. Xavier Crement, *A**hole No More!: A Self-Help Guide for Recovering A**holes* (Canal Winchester, OH: Enthea Press, 1991).

17. Video cameras have become so inexpensive and easy-to-use that you can make your own videos. Be a director: tape your Swell-Wimp workouts!

18. To be more precise, the results are almost the same. Women do not lose as much weight as men in the short term (15–30 minutes) but their long-term results are the same. See Appendix A.

19. For more on this see George Tylutki, "What Good is *self?*" *Computer Language*, May 1989, 34–47.

20. Hard work and will power succeed. [ed.]

21. *Everything You Always Wanted To Know About Sex But Were Afraid To Ask* (NY: Bantam Books, 1969).

22. See Walter A. Brown, "The Placebo Effect," *Scientific American*, January 1998, 90–95 for more on the importance of having faith in Swell-Wimp.

23. The Institute for Writing and Thinking at Bard College held a workshop titled "Teaching Emily Dickinson" in April 1994. The course description states "Emily Dickinson is often characterized as an eccentric recluse who meditated upon death— a shy, fearful woman who withdrew from the world. ...This workshop questions the conventional view of Emily Dickinson through a close reading of the poet's less well-known poems that reveal a strongly metaphysical perspective and a mystical sensibility." As my niece might say, "Well, duh!" Even first-year literature students know that about one-third of her poems are about death, one-third about nature and one-third about other topics. Apparently the "Institute" hasn't been doing much "Thinking" about Dickinson; there is no mention of her sexual experimentation nor even her erotic poetry. See Appendix B for the skinny on the "eccentric recluse."

24. The poems attributed to Dickinson ("The Dove Bar," "The Triumph," and "Sominex") by Mark O'Donnell in his book *Vertigo Park* (NY: Alfred A. Knopf, 1993) were not written by her; they are pure invention. She did not work as a copy-

writer for an advertising agency in Boston. Sominex hadn't even been invented while she was alive! You must be constantly vigilant for this kind of shoddy scholarship.

25. Acquiring new habits and breaking old patterns is difficult even when the alternative is superior. For example, the Dvorak keyboard, which enables you to type much more quickly and with less effort, has not replaced the Qwerty keyboard. Chevalier d'Eon, who wrote *Menage a trois—Why not?* (Boston: Coituphilous Publications, 1972), was also the inventor of the Tribow which enables a violinist to play three-note chords instead of only two-note chords. Despite its superiority it has not caught on probably because it is unwieldy and requires the acquisition of an entirely different bowing technique.

26. Swell-Wimp is appropriate for older people. See Chapter 14.

27. The term "feedback," originally derived from electronics, refers to the return (feeding back) of a portion of a signal to a circuit in order to maintain the output. **Feed**back is an unfortunate term when applied to a weight-loss program, as is its association with loud noise (a microphone/amplifier loop). However, see Chapter 6.

28. Kinsey in *Sexual Behavior in the Human Male* writes, "On the whole it is evident that general good health and, therefore, the physical activity which engenders good health, may contribute to an increase in the frequency of sexual performance" (Philadelphia and London: W. B. Saunders, 1948, 206).

29. For more on impotence, see Chapter 14.

30. This is exactly what happened with one of the study participants, Mr. Norbert.

31. It is generally assumed that TB is a disease of the past—that we have eradicated it—but this is not true. The incidence of TB infection has risen sharply in recent years, primarily because of drug users who do not take their medicine, remain infectious and spread the disease to others. There has even appeared a form of TB that is resistant to the cheap and readily-available antibiotics used to cure TB patients.

32. Yes, this sounds like the ridiculous logic of many political conservatives who argue for giving the police more power by saying that an innocent person should not be afraid to answer police questions. They fail to understand (1) that police do make mistakes; (2) innocence is a relative state; (3) certain rights are absolute; (4) constitutional safeguards are meant to protect the innocent as well as the guilty; and (5) a bigger gun (more power) never solves a problem. But getting an exam is easy and will confirm your opinion and reassure your partner.

33. "Straight Sex and AIDS Vaccines," *Discover*, Jan 1992.

34. Even some priests and archbishops are more sexually active than the average man or woman, and although your partner may be a judge or legislator, you cannot be sure he is AIDS-free. C. F.

35. Some people must now consent to an medical examination to keep their jobs and to get insurance. Probably even more will have to in the future. Statistically, as more tests are done, more mistakes will be made. So get an exam now and avoid the rush and thus the increased possibility of faulty results.

36. *Caveat emptor* reversed.

37. As William Thackery writes in *Vanity Fair* (1848: Harmondsworth, Middlesex, England: Penguin Books, 1968), 663: "Be gentle with those who are less lucky, if not more deserving. Think, what right have you to be scornful, whose virtue is a deficiency of temptation, whose success may be a chance, whose rank may be an ancestor's accident, whose prosperity is very likely a satire."

38. You may find it fruitful to read *I Hope* (trans. David Floyd) by Raisa Maksimovna Titorenko, another researcher who strongly hoped (Harper Collins, 1991).

Chapter 2

1. Some researchers believe that a molecule called neuropeptide Y (NPY) may cause some people to overeat. It is a neurotransmitter, a small protein that carries signals between nerve cells in the brain. When NPY is given to rats, they overeat. Researchers at the University of California at Riverside have tested an antiserum to NPY and when injected into normal rats the animals ate about 60% less than usual even when deprived of food before the injection. This antiserum will not be the diet drug of the future because antibodies can't cross the blood-brain barrier, but researchers hope to develop a drug that blocks the receptor sites of NPY on nerve cells. ("The Brain of a Glutton," *Discover*, June 1992, 14–15).

2. Nordic Trac advertisement, *The New Yorker*, September 2, 1991, 69.

3. Moderate exercise is any exercise equivalent to thirty to sixty minutes of brisk walking each day.

4. Unfortunately, we cannot convert the sun's energy into a form usable by our bodies (photosynthesis) as plants do.

5. Some might argue that sexual intercourse is an activity necessary to maintain life in the sense that without intercourse there would be no life. It could also be said that intercourse is an activity necessary to maintain life to some people, in that without sex they would not want to live. Some might even say that if they couldn't bowl (or swim or read) they would die. But, by life-maintaining activities we mean prima-

rily the autonomous or involuntary body activities: heart pumping, lungs inhaling and exhaling, etc.

6. See Appendix A for a description of the opposition we encountered.

7. In *Consumer Reports* (November 1993, 729–733), Consumers Union concludes that the home gyms they tested could "build strength and tone muscles," but "none bowled us over." They go on to say that "there are other ways to reap the benefits a home gym provides," and briefly discuss four alternatives: free weights, bands and springs, health clubs and aerobic exercise. There is no mention of Swell-Wimp! Consumers Union has an excellent reputation for fairness and objectivity, but in this case it is clear that some sort of institutional prejudice prevented them from even considering sexual exercise as an alternative.

8. Also, sex was seen as an unequal, bilateral activity in which the male was active and the female passive. Thus, the female's role was seen as barely physical. The male had to be vigorous FOR sex; he didn't become vigorous BECAUSE of sex. C. F.

9. However, see Chapter 13, note 1.

10. It is often said by coaches, drill instructors and fathers that *quae nocent docent* (things that hurt teach), although not in Latin. This kind of learning should be avoided during SexAct.

11. January 1998, 60. They also say that "the road to weight loss is more likely to start with a trip to the bookstore—not the pharmacy [for diet pills]," so tell your friends that CP recommends reading our book.

12. Wardell Pomeroy, a leading sexologist, often asks an audience to think of a four-letter word ending in "k" that means "intercourse." The word that he means is "talk." The term "intercourse" has come to be associated almost solely with sexual activity. It can be (and was in the past) applied to many interactions, such as social intercourse and verbal intercourse. Another term whose definition has narrowed is "prophylactic" which has come to mean only a condom (a noun), although the term may also be a modifier (taking an aspirin as a prophylactic measure). Another example of a word whose common definition has narrowed: in Charles Dickens' *Bleak House* Sir Leicester "leans back in his chair, and breathlessly ejaculates"; however, what he ejaculates is not semen but "Good heaven!" (Penguin Books, 1971, 781).

13. By sex we mean sexual activity which is actions involving the sex organs and their functions whose purpose is procreation and/or erotic pleasure. We do not mean a symbolic-expression or S-expression, which in Lisp (a computer language developed by John McCarthy in 1958; see also Franz Lisp, "Hungarian Notation," *Programmer's Update*, July 1990, 18–35) is an atom or a dotted pair where each element of the pair is a Sex (see *Byte*, November 1991, 165 for more information).

14. Coitus is a term derived from Latin that means sexual intercourse between human beings.

15. As you probably know, *Caveat emptor* means "buyer beware" and *caveat venditor* means "seller beware." However, "caveat" is not a verb even though politicians use it that way: "I think we need to caveat that recommendation."

16. For more about changing attitudes, see Chapter 14.

17. Nothing we say in this book could disturb the social fabric as much as the activities of a person in Congress during a single term. C. F.

18. You have probably heard of the Spur Posse—a clique of middle-class boys in California, who kept a competitive count of how many girls they had bedded and fondled. You shouldn't compete when the activities are pleasurable. As soon as it becomes competitive, it ceases to be fun (golfing or swimming for money). Imagine competing with your friends to see who could listen to the most symphonies or eat the most cheesecake or read the greatest number of Emily Dickinson poems. The pressures of competition force one to do unpleasurable, even unpleasant, things one wouldn't do otherwise (think lawyer); the boys admitted to fondling girls as young as ten and to having encounters with girls they did not find attractive simply to up their tallies. P. B.

Those boys were social and moral, if not legal, criminals. They gave no attention to the responsibilities of sexual activity. They didn't care who they hurt. Let's hope they transmitted no diseases to their "partners." C. F.

19. Also called the Cowper's glands. See note 2, Chapter 4.

20. Incidentally, Swell-Wimp is unrelated to astronomical WIMP (Weakly Interacting Massive Particles) which are thought by some to comprise galactic halos.

21. Relativism concerning sexual matters is not new: Vatsyayana, the author of the *Kama Sutra*, writing between the first and fourth century AD, points out that what is normal or permissible concerning sexual conduct in one place may be considered vice in another.

22. In the prologue to the Miller's Tale Chaucer points out that the tales are "bettre or werse" (and the Miller's is worse), but he must repeat them as he heard them "Or elles falsen som of my mateere." Therefore, if the reader is easily offended, he (or she) should "Turne over the leef and chese another tale;/ For he shal fynde ynowe, grete and smale,/ Of storial thyng that toucheth gentillesse,/ and eek moralitee and hoolynesse./ Blameth nat me if that ye chese amys./ .../ Avyseth yow, and put me out of blame" (*The Tales of Canterbury*, ed. Robert A. Pratt [Boston: Houghton Mifflin, 1974], ll. 3171–3185).

23. Boccaccio says, "those who read these tales can leave those they dislike and read those they like. I do not want to deceive anybody, and so all these tales bear written at the head a title explaining what they contain" (*The Decameron*, trans. Richard Aldington [NY: Dell, 1930], 639).

24. Activities such as those held by several aging United States Senators, who, unable to understand the methods and aims of our research, seem to be trying to prevent us from receiving funding from the Federal Government. *Damnant quod non intelligunt.*[a] These are the same men who wouldn't allow the discussion of sex in relation to AIDS in federally-funded programs and materials if the materials offended "community standards." So, you can see the type of people we have to deal with. During the Bush administration, a cartoon by Lowe in the Fort Lauderdale *Sun-Sentinel* summed things up. In the first pane the Center for Disease Control (CDC) is being told that it can't mention condoms in its AIDS education campaign. In the second panel we see a man and woman listening to a CDC speaker: "So, don't forget to put on your **MITTENS** before you look under the **CABBAGE LEAF!**" Still, we hope to be able to continue our studies in the near future.

25. At least not in terms of weight loss and fitness.

26. *Sexual Behavior in the Human Male* (Philadelphia and London: W. B. Saunders, 1948), 325.

27. In Chapter 7 we discuss hair and shaving at greater length.

28. Any sexual activity that results in orgasm should correlate closely to intercourse in regards to energy expenditure. However, there are differences that prevent making any claims for these practices without further research.

29. In Poem 577 Emily Dickinson writes approvingly about necrophilia; however, we have been unable to find any evidence that she ever actually engaged in this practice:

> For tho' they lock Thee in the Grave,
> Myself—can own the key—
> Think of it Lover! I and Thee
> Permitted—face to face to be—
> Forgive me, if to stroke thy frost
> Outvisions Paradise!

30. Kinsey reports that about 6% of the total male population has been involved in animal contacts of some sort during early adolescence (*Sexual Behavior in the Human Male*, 262) and that 1.5% of females had some sort of sexual relations with

animals in pre-adolescence and 3.6% after adolescence (*Sexual Behavior in the Human Female*, 505).

31. Dickinson experimented with bondage with a telegraph operator; apparently she liked it (Poem 725):

> What Thou dost—is Delight—
> Bondage as Play—be sweet—
> Just We two...
> What Thou dost not—Despair

32. An excellent book, *The Poo Perplex* has been written about this by Frederick Crews (NY: NAL-Dutton, 1965).

33. Nor will we be discussing anal intercourse because: (1) in terms of energy expenditure, it differs only slightly from rear-mount (doggie style) intercourse; (2) anal intercourse can damage delicate internal tissues (the rectum was not designed to be battered by an erect penis or any other penis-like device); (3) it is nasty-dirty. Don't touch.

34. This is a good place to point out that if you engage in (love) biting, you should be careful not to do so at or near orgasm. During orgasm, the jaws go into spasm and can bite really hard. Therefore, you should never climax with a penis, breast or finger in your mouth.

35. See Chapter 7, *Kama Sutra* where he discusses the various modes of striking and of the sounds appropriate to them.

36. Besides, it would be impossible to obtain funding to continue our research if we were to include these activities in our study.

37. For example, Ken Eichenbaum's *The Toilets of New York* (Milwaukee: Litterati Books, 1991) contains 100 detailed descriptions of men's and women's toilets and this could be very useful, especially to tourists. However, the title is misleading; the book does not cover New York state, nor even New York city. It covers Manhattan only!

38. K. Heslinga says 97% of boys and 35% of girls masturbate (112).

39. Unfortunately, not everyone is comfortable with this. Shere Hite reports that most women she interviewed said they enjoyed masturbation physically and many saw it as a means of independence from men and a means to better sex, but many had psychological problems with it because they felt that it was dirty or selfish or something only an unattractive and lonely person would do (6–13). For a full discussion of the development of the belief that masturbation is harmful, see K. Heslinga, *Not Made of Stone* (Springfield, Illinois: Charles C. Thomas, 1974).

40. See Galway Kinnell, *When One has Lived a Long Time Alone* (NY: Knopf, 1991) and Richard E. Byrd, *Alone* (NY: G. P. Putnam's Sons, 1938).

41. *Sexual Behavior in the Human Female*, 132. 62% of all females had masturbated at some time in their lives and 58% had masturbated to the point of orgasm. 45% reached orgasm in 3 minutes or less and 25% in 4 to 5 minutes.

42. A new infinitive apparently.

43. For more on "dildonics" (his term) see Don Lancaster, "The ISMM Revisited (II)," *Midnight Engineering*, Sep/Oct 1991, 62.

44. You don't want to look like a professional tennis player with one upper quadrant overdeveloped. Or maybe you do.

45. *On Sex and Human Loving* (Boston & Toronto: Little, Brown and Co., 1982), 59. They note that the myotonia is often visible in the facial muscles where a grimace or frown may be seen (72). Therefore, a smile of bliss or pleasure on your partner's face is often an indication that he or she is "faking it."

46. See Chapter 5 concerning sexual energy expenditure and teasing.

Chapter 3

1. Life is not being alive but being well. [ed.]

2. *Sexual Behavior in the Human Male* (Philadelphia and London: W. B. Saunders, 1948), 193–197. They consider the following as types of sexual outlet: masturbation, nocturnal emissions, heterosexual petting, heterosexual intercourse, homosexual relations, and intercourse with animals. They found that there are eleven factors of primary importance in determining the frequency and sources of human sexual outlet: sex, race, age, age at onset of adolescence, marital status, educational level, occupational class, parent's occupational class, rural-urban background, religious affiliation and extent of devotion to religious affairs.

3. *Sexual Behavior in the Human Female*, (Philadelphia and London: W. B. Saunders, 1953), 349.

4. *The New Joy of Sex* (New York: Crown Publishers, 1991); *Everything You Always Wanted to Know About Sex* (NY: Bantam Books, 1969).

5. *New York Magazine*, December 8, 1972 in *The Book of Lists*, David Wallenchinsky, Irving Wallace and Amy Wallace (NY: Bantam Books, 1977).

6. See Chapter 10, note 30.

7. Colman McCarthy, "The Politics of Bicycling," *Liberal Opinion Week*, 28 December 1992.

8. Of course, you must first have a complete physical examination: sex will not be cheap if you are hospitalized for a heart attack. Nor will it be cheap if you contract a venereal disease because you did not choose your partner carefully. Nor will it be cheap if you are arrested for passing on a communicable disease (as can happen in some jurisdictions). See also Chapter 9.

9. Everyone should wear a helmet **and** mirror (it clips onto your glasses or helmet) while riding a bicycle. Forget the fancy biking pants and shoes and spend your money on safety: a well-dressed corpse is...dead!

10. Of course, if you hire a sexual partner it may not be cheaper, depending upon the average service charge in your area, the price of bicycles and greens fees. Some of you may find it necessary to hire a partner and this can inhibit spontaneity somewhat. Emily Dickinson was not above accepting payment for sex (Poem 580):

> I gave myself to Him—
> And took Himself, for Pay,
> At least—'tis Mutual— Risk—
> Some— found it— Mutual Gain—
> Sweet Debt of Life— Each Night to owe—
> Insolvent— every Noon—

Incidentally, if you do hire a partner, you should avoid organizations that urge you to charge the fees to your employer's credit card; he or she won't like it (unless you are your employer) and neither will the police.

11. In this book we do not discuss group-sex. If you are really serious about losing weight or getting fit, you will not depend upon group-sex activities as a primary method. The difficulties of arranging sessions can make it difficult to keep to any kind of schedule. Also you are much more likely to be injured or get sick if you have sex in a group (even children get more colds during the school year because they spend their days in groups). The emotional-psychological interactions between two sexual partners are complex and delicate. Among many partners they become a dangerous tangled web which threatens the psychological-emotional health of all. Thus, we advise against group sex, at least until we are able to conduct more studies and publish our findings.

12. Lawrence Schiller, in "Justice Boulder Style" (*The New Yorker*, 19 Jan. 1998, 32-37), profiles a District Attorney who "recently passed the eighteen-thousand-mile mark on his Schwinn exercycle" (36). An announcement that a person has washed

249,000 dishes or taken 1863 rectal temperatures is a statement about honest, useful, remunerative work. But 18,000 miles on an exercycle! How many mind-numbing, arse-numbing hours is that? C. F.

13. It seems to me that stationary bicycles, treadmills and other similar devices could be designed to run generators as the users operated them so as to recharge batteries, especially laptop computer batteries. The users would gain a greater sense of accomplishment (as well as an exercise goal) and countless kilowatts of energy might be saved. C. F.

14. If you must drive, at least, use a manual shift car with hand-cranked windows.

15. We will have nothing to say about the Lewinsky matter; it would be like shooting fish in a barrel.

16. From *Arms Amatoria*: Dumbbells keep dumbbells busy.

17. It has been pointed out that such a recommendation may be a conflict of interests or at least made in our own self-interest since increasing the number of Swell-Wimp participants means a greater number of copies of this book being sold. That may be true. But the recommendation was made in regards to the government where self-interest rules and conflicts of interest are ignored.

18. *The Economic Factor and the Health of Sex Professionals* (Detroit: Ouslan Press, 1977). Sélavy and Taque studied the health of women who made their living by illegally engaging in sexual activities (whores, prostitutes, trollops, harlots, strumpets, and street walkers but not sex therapists or sex surrogates). Basically, they found that the more the women charged, the more likely they were to be healthy. For example, call girls were much healthier than street prostitutes. One item they used to measure the health of the women was their weight. See also James Plunkett's *Strumpet City* (NY: Dell, 1969) and *Trollope* by N. John Hall (Oxford University Press, 1991).

19. A similar study by Drs. Popadià Pope and Athole Athwiper, *National Health Care and the Self-Employed* (Thule: Boinkmeister, 1986) studied Eastern European prostitutes and came to similar preliminary conclusions (the study was not completed due to political unrest in the area). Interestingly only 62% of the whores studied would have been within 3% of their ideal weight by American standards. This is due to poorer diets (more underweight subjects) and cultural attitudes about what is healthy- and sexy-looking (more "overweight" subjects). Still, 89% of the harlots studied weighed less than the average female in these countries. See also, Anna Leonoweng, *The Romance of the Harem*, Susan Morgan ed. (Charlottesville: University Press of Virginia, 1991).

20. You have been warned. Don't tell your physician that Bathous and Flanders said it was OK to have sex as much as you like!

21. Foreplay, postplay, and diet are equally important whether you engage in FreqSex or StrenSex.

22. Our favorite poet apparently didn't mind the wait (Poem 781):

> To wait an Hour— is long—
> If Love be just beyond—
> To wait Eternity— is short—
> If Love reward the end

However, you should probably postpone sexual activity after a heavy meal since the partner on the bottom might become sick.

23. The Romans called this *a mensa et toro*, "from table to bed."

24. See Alfredo E. de Newman's book, *Quid? Perturbabo?* (Arco, Idaho: Kycarsius and Co., 1987) for more about developing bilateral commitments.

25. Everything in moderation. [ed.]

Chapter 4

1. Quoted in "The Healing Powers of Sex," by Kristin von Kreisler in *Reader's Digest*, June 1993, 18; reprinted from *Redbook*, April 1993.

2. As William Cowper said, "Variety's the very spice of life" (*The Task*, "The Timepiece," 1. 606).

3. "The Pima Paradox, *The New Yorker*, 2 Feb. 1998, 44–57. Gladwell's article discusses the Pima Indian tribe which is the fattest group of people in the world except for the Nauru Islanders of the West Pacific.

4. Von Kreisler, 18.

5. Even after allowing for different body masses, Von Kreisler's rates of 8 calories per minute for women and 12 for men indicate that he makes an unwarranted assumption about the degree of activity of the female. C. F.

6. But, there are pockets of ignorance. If this idea (that women can and should enjoy sex and be an equal partner in the activity) is new to you, then we recommend that you read one of the following books: *The Hite Report* by Shere Hite, *Lesbia Brandon* by A. C. Swinburne (London: Falcon Press, 1952), *The Feminine Mystique* by Betty Friedan (NY: Norton, 1963), *Motherlines* by Suzy McKee Charnas (NY: Berkley Publishing, 1978), *Kalogynomia: or the Laws of Female Beauty* by T. Bell (London: J. J. Stockdale, 1821), *Purely for Pleasure* by Margaret Lane (London: H.

Hamilton, 1966), *Herland* by Charlotte Perkins Gilman (NY: Pantheon Books, 1979), *This Side of Paradise* by Francis S. Fitzgerald (NY: A. L. Burt, 1920), *Liberal Imagination* by L. Trilling (Garden City, NY: Doubleday, 1953), and *The Female Eunuch* by Germaine Greer (London: MacGibbon & Kee, 1970).

7. As John Payne Collier said, *"Stod solidus cedilla; aigu breve hacek!"*

8. For example, checking the oil in your car, paying bills on time, buttoning all of your buttons and zipping all of your zippers.

9. *Extra!*, March/April 1999, 22–24.

10. For example, tracking average monthly electricity usage, counting the sheets of toilet paper as you use it, and refusing to turn the TV on until seconds before a show begins.

Chapter 5

1. During sexual arousal, most people display unusual muscular strength and exhibit muscular contractions (and relaxations) from head to toe. Kinsey, Pomeroy, Martin and Gebhard in *Sexual Behavior in the Human Female* (Philadelphia & London: W. B. Saunders, 1953) report that some partial paraplegics may be improved when they are sexually aroused. Apparently some mechanism is at work that enables them to control some muscles that they cannot when not sexually aroused. It should be noted that the control is not so extensive or specific that a paraplegic would want to maintain a state of sexual arousal in order to improve mobility.

2. The carpopedal spasm in which the big toe is held straight out while the other toes bend back and the foot arches.

3. Dickinson in Poem 393 lamented the brevity of orgasm:

> Did [If] Our Best Moment last—
> 'Twould supersede the Heaven—
> These Heavenly Moments are—
> A Grant of the Divine—
> That Certain as it Comes—
> Withdraws…

4. Ejaculation is not the same thing as orgasm. Both men and women have orgasms, but only men ejaculate and some men have orgasms without ejaculation.

5. The French terms "La petite mort" (the little death) and "La mort douce" (the sweet death) refer to the syncope that sometimes occurs at the moment of climax. P. B.

Well, this rarely happens. Fainting by women during orgasm is primarily a myth invented by men as evidence of their sexual power. This myth of women's frailty also proved useful to some women as a means of avoiding intercourse with brutish husbands. C. F.

6. Thus, it is mandatory that you have a complete physical examination before beginning Swell-Wimp! Since health care is a for-profit enterprise in the United States, it may be difficult for some of you to afford an examination. This is unfortunate, but you should not begin Swell-Wimp unless you are sure you are healthy enough to do so. We commend President Clinton for trying to bring about some sort of health-care reform, but his plan would have made a bad system only slightly less bad. For-profit health care can never be universal, complete or inexpensive. Radical reform is needed, not more regulations to keep the greedy from becoming exceedingly rich. Many people complain that the government cannot

7. do anything right, and thus a government-run health-care system would be inefficient and expensive. Would they abolish the Social Security system and privatize the military? It is usually these same conservatives who praise the US military (a government program) as the best in the world. They complain that the public schools are a disgrace but claim that our higher-education system is the best in the world. Don't they realize that they are comparing apples and oranges. Neither the military nor the universities are required to accept everyone and deliver basic services to everyone and both can simply throw out anyone who fails to meet their standards (behavioral, social, moral, educational, etc.). Change the public schools' mandate; allow them to eject the troublemakers, at least the incorrigibles (as private schools can), and you'd see an amazing improvement in the schools in a short time. Even when there was a draft and the military was forced to accept everyone, it could still discharge or imprison anyone who failed to meet its standards. Public schools, the military and private education simply cannot be compared. But the problems in public education are not the topic of this note. "They" say that the health-care system is in bad shape, but also claim that "we" have the best health-care in the world, for those who can afford it. Doesn't there seem to be an analogy here to education? The two systems (health care and public education)—one based on local property taxes (the stupidest scheme in the world) and the other on pay-as-you-go fees—fail to provide basic services to everyone. Isn't it obvious that

8. if we funded health-care and public education as we do the military, we would be able to provide the best health care in the world to every citizen? Of course, it

would be very expensive, as is national defense. The interstate highway system was built only after it was declared that such a system was necessary to national security. Every person in Congress has schools and health-care facilities in his or her district (as they do military-related facilities). They should have no problems declaring health and education to be national (not local) concerns and as important as national defense. If we must waste tax money, let us "waste" it on developing an educated, healthy citizenry. Wouldn't we rather export health-care and education than export arms? Some things must be strictly regulated, funded and administered at the national level, not left to market forces. Of course, any rational, comprehensive health-care plan would help people pay for those things they might need for Swell-Wimp.

9. Of all of the photographs of a couple making love in *The New Joy of Sex* by Alex Comfort (NY: Crown Publishers, 1991), not one shows a penis, although several show the woman's pubic area and most show her breasts. Comfort's "Gourmet Guide to Lovemaking" seems not to approve of showing what A. A. Milne calls "Binker" in "Bathtime," *Now We Are Six*. C. F.

10. Historically, males have made virtues of their limitations, but since that failed to convince women that they were superior (and even failed to convince many men), they simply dominated women. Most women have desired men for what they could offer—a little pleasure, some financial security and children. And they have feared men in varying degrees. Every woman with an ounce of sensitivity has felt sadness for and anger toward men—limited, dominating dolts, without the innocence of children but with the same self-centerdness and lack of control. The conflicting emotions of desire and fear and anger and sadness resulted in women remaining subordinate. Today, there is no reason to fear men in general (in developed nations) and the anger has found outlets (in the courts, for example). So, an intelligent woman is more likely to feel only desire and sadness. Since the desire can be satisfied regularly, sadness dominates.

Some women find that they are overcome with sadness; they become depressed (and depression feeds depression). There is no denying that there is much to be sad about regarding men, but their situation is partly biological and partly their own doing (for thousands of years). Yes, it is better to feel sadness for men than to feel as they did and often do: superior to and contemptuous of women. However, sadness can be transformed to concern and to caring actions and, as Emily Dickinson says, you may even "Love the dull lad" (Poem 267). C. F.

11. For example, Juliet says, "Stay but a little, I will come again" (*Romeo and Juliet*, 2:2:44). William H. Masters, Virginia E. Johnson and Robert C. Kolodny, *On Sex and Human Loving* (Boston & Toronto: Little, Brown and Co., 1982) describe

four levels for the sexual response cycle: excitement or arousal, plateau, orgasm and resolution.

12. Although almost all women have the potential to be multi-orgasmic, Kinsey, Pomeroy, Martin and Gebhard in *Sexual Behavior in the Human Female*, note that only 14% of females report achieving multiple orgasm regularly (375). SexAct should not be thought of as what one woman calls the "The Orgasm Olympics." If you achieve multiple orgasm, that's great. If you don't, you might want to try modifying your techniques so that you can. If you don't, that's OK. If you don't achieve orgasm at all, you should do something about it. See the next section.

13. Nobody knows how many orgasms a woman can have, but David Reuben in *Everything You Always Wanted to Know About Sex* But Were Afraid to Ask (NY: Bantam Books, 1969) reports that fifty consecutive orgasms have been recorded.

14. Of course, every orgasm of a multiple orgasmic experience may not be mind-blowing. Some are intense and some are mild (so much so that her partner may not even know that she is experiencing one). The male orgasm also ranges from intense to mild.

15. Thus, there arose the myth of the nymphomaniac. Because men must recharge after climax and because they recharge more slowly as they age, men concluded that a women who likes and wants sex and who could enjoy it more frequently than they must be disturbed. Ironically many men dream of an encounter with one of these crazy women. Nymphomania is also called the Messalina Complex. The term is derived from the "notorious" female, Messalina, the wife of the Roman Emperor Claudius, who had sexual encounters with numerous men, supposedly because of her insatiable appetite for sexual intercourse. Men called her disturbed, but it is more likely that she had difficulty finding "a noble Roman" who could bring her to climax. C. F.

16. You should note also that males cannot lose much weight simply from ejaculating. Of course, an ounce or more of semen is expelled but this is mostly fluid and the body immediately begins to replenish it. Repeated frequent ejaculation (10 to 20 times a day) will result in diminishing the amount of semen ejaculated each time, causing you to become very thirsty and probably sore. Any loss of weight will be regained within twenty-four hours.

17. Thus, we might say that women are more environmentally friendly; they recycle more quickly than men. As Robert Burns writes: "Auld Nature swears, the lovely dears/ Her noblest work she classes, O:/ Her prentice han' she try'd on man,/ An' then she made the lasses, O" ("Epistle to a Young Friend" [1786]). C. F.

18. Women sometimes experience depression because of the knowledge that they have control of their sexual apparatus in a way and to a degree that males do not. The poor male can't do much more than "get it up" and push it back and forth. Males are so helpless. They have so little control. They can get erections during sleep and even under anesthesia, yet getting it up and keeping it up are not guaranteed at any given time even for "virile" men. After they achieve climax, they are almost always immediately rendered impotent for a while (although, possibly unfortunately, not in the same manner or degree as male rabbits). And they can recycle and achieve orgasm only two or three times a night (despite their bragging). Their sexual organs are so exposed and vulnerable to injury and embarrassment (erections at inappropriate times; the bane of male adolescents). And, of course, they can do no more than "spread their seed." It is the female who receives the seed and produces (and nurtures) the baby. Although sensitivity to the male's plight is good, you should not let it depress you; that will not do you or your partner any good. C. F.

Dr. Flanders overstates the case, but I certainly agree with her last sentence. P. B.

I don't overstate the case; men simply lack control. For example, they can become aroused and ejaculate in their sleep. If this happened to women, it would be considered further evidence of their irrational, emotional nature. But in men it is regarded as normal and simply called "nocturnal emissions." C. F.

Women also can become aroused and climax while sleeping. P. B.

True, but much less frequently and we don't "emit" all over the sheets. C. F.

Uncle. P. B.

19. There is a sensuous spot just above the buttocks called *chute de reins*. It is easier to find on fat people because back fat produced dimples at this point. It is worth searching for this spot; simultaneously you can rub the lower back (where a lot of tension accumulates) relaxing the muscles and increasing blood flow to the area and arouse your partner (or yourself).

20. The exercises were named after their inventor, Arnold Kegel, who was a surgeon. They are often used during pregnancy to help facilitate delivery and postpartum to help the vagina regain its shape and fitness. See Chapter 8 for more information about using Kegel exercises for strengthening the vaginal muscles.

21. Not with your fingers in your vagina, of course.

22. William Butler Yeats writes in "Crazy Jane Talks With The Bishop":

> Fair and foul are near of kin,
> And fair needs foul...
>
> ....

> But Love has pitched his mansion in
> The place of excrement;
> For nothing can be sole or whole
> That has not been rent.

And in Jonathan Swift's "The Lady's Dressing Room," the speaker asks "Should I the Queen of Love refuse,/ Because she rose from stinking Ooze?" and answers no, because "Such Order from Confusion sprung,/ Such gaudy Tulips rais'd from Dung" (ll. 131–32, 143–44). However, in Swift's "Cassinus and Peter," Cassinus is driven to distraction: "Nor wonder how I lost my Wits;/ Oh! *Caelia, Caelia Caelia* sh—"(ll. 117–8).

23. Alex Comfort says that women have two mouths: one on her face and one between her legs (the vulva). He notes that many men are afraid of the vulva: it looks like a castration wound, it bleeds regularly, it swallows the erect penis, and regurgitates it limp (52). Might this fear account, in part, for the subjugation of women by men? C. F.

24. Dr. Bathous informs me that "poop" means tush. It is a regionalism used in phrases such as "soft as a baby's poop." C. F.

25. It will take some practice before you are be able to pedal, work the handlebars back and forth and roll your head simultaneously. However, it is unlikely that you will fall off and, once mastered, this technique will enable you to warm up quickly and efficiently.

26. Many people find it easier to do head rolls while rowing, probably because they are closer to the floor (and thus are less afraid of falling) and because the seats on rowing machines are larger and thus the exerciser is more stable.

27. Those of you who are nudists are already aware of these aspects. We recommend that you warm up partially or fully clothed, since it is the change in clothedness that yields the psychological benefits.

28. Dr. Bathous overstates the case, but I certainly agree that naked warm-ups can be arousing. C. F.

29. See *Wild Desire* by Karen Brennan (Univ. of Mass. Press, 1991).

30. Dickinson writes of the pleasures of foreplay in Poem 391:

> Who visits in the Night—
> And just before the Sun—
> Caresses—and is gone—
> But whom his fingers touched—
> And whatsoever Mouth he kissed—
> Is as it had not been—

31. *The Hite Report* (NY: Macmillan; London: Collier Macmillan, 1976), 178.

32. Dickinson had a related problem. She experienced extremely pleasurable orgasms and reacted with violent motions, so much so that they interfered with her partner's orgasm. She writes of this in Poem 218: "I shouldn't like to come/ For fear of joggling Him!"

33. I'm told that *The 5,000 Fingers of Dr. T.* by Theodore Geisel is an excellent how-to manual (it's also available on video, which I plan to review soon).

34. See Pauline Kael's excellent 1968 how-to manual *Kiss Kiss, Bang Bang* (Boston: Little Brown, 1968). Did you know that in Slovakian a "smooch" is a ski?

35. Thus, wearing heavy earrings contributes to a continued sensual experience for many women, especially if they rub against the neck.

36. In fact, many are put off by the sight. For example, in Thomas Hardy's *The Mayor of Casterbridge* (Boston: Houghton Mifflin, 1962), Mrs. Mayor "beheld the unattractive exterior of Farfrae's erection" and became disgusted (89).

37. Well, voyeurs are usually male. C. F.

Of cours, and, therefore, strippers are usually women. P. B.

38. We recommend Magritte's *Le principe de plaisir* and anything from his 1947 *fauve* (*vache*) period. We especially like Rabo Karabekian's 1987 painting *Now It's Women's Turn*. Although many people find Ralph Albert Blakelock's *Forest Scene with Brook* perplexing, we believe that it can stimulate us at the beginning of SexEx (foreplay) to be attentive to the fact that many things go into making a beautiful, lasting experience. Many of Balthasar Klossowski's works are appropriate. Also nice are Marilyn Minter's "Food Porn" works. A reproduction of Juan Carreño de Miranda's *La Monstrua* reminds you of what you are trying to avoid and its reds brighten up a room.

39. Kinsey, *Sexual Behavior in Females*, 651–664. See also Chapters 6, 13 and 10.

40. Or possibly "Fourplay"; we have been unable to find any of their recordings in the campus store.

41. Michael Vestey reported on this broadcast for *The Spectator* (27 March 1999, 51–52), titling his piece "Decent Into Tackiness." We disagree. There might be more stations playing classical music if they responded to their listeners' needs and preferences as this one did (nothing is more stimulating than good music).

42. Adam Phillips in *Kissing, Tickling and Being Bored* (Cambridge, Mass: Harvard University Press, 1993) discusses this technique.

43. They also prohibit non-contact dancing because the gyrations of the dancers are considered obscene and arousing also.

44. See Chapter 10 for more about dancing during intercourse.

45. Sexual Behavior in Females, 364.

46. One could easily argue that unmarried couples spend more or less time in foreplay. Since they often do not have the same time pressures (where are the kids?) and suffer less from boredom due to years of intimacy, they might conduct their sexual encounters leisurely. On the other hand, since the group of unmarried couples is composed of prostitutes and their clients, lawyers between courtroom appearances, and teenagers, it is just as likely that they do not spend more time on foreplay.

47. For more on frigidity, see Chapter 14.

48. Shere Hite reports that many women in her survey said that extended arousal during foreplay felt good, but that many men wouldn't wait for very long. Clearly, sex is not much fun if the man goes on to climax leaving the woman with no orgasm (68–70). C. F.

Chapter 6

1. Erotic talk.

2. Vatsyayana in Chapter 3 of *Kama Sutra* discusses the various sounds made at the "time of union" and acknowledges that when the sounds are made is unimportant. He does not, however, deal with the sounds in terms of energy expenditure or their appropriateness or ease of use. Also see Val and Tina Rudolf, *The Shrieking Chic Sheik* (Stercoraceous, NY: Sirreverence Books, 1923).

3. They are quieter than fish. [ed.]

4. He (or she) who remains silent consents. [bob]

5. Or someone. C. F.

6. Possibly literally. C. F.

7. You should probably avoid macaronic verse and the poetry of the German poet Michael Hamburger. (Just a little joke. P. B.)

8. Mentioning their mothers, wives or former lovers.

9. An excessive flow of words analogous to diarrhea. Unlike *cacoëthes loquendi* for which there is no cure, the medication Thoro Zeptate or a half pound of cheese will relieve the symptoms of logorrhea. Amazingly, the Amazonian Kayapó tribe has 23 different words for diarrhea and none for logorrhea.

10. This is not to say that biting and nail-scratching have not and do not play a role in sexual activities. Vatsyayana devotes considerable space in the *Kama Sutra* (Chapter 4) to this subject and says that nothing tends to increase "love" so much as

the effects of marking with the nails and biting. John Cleland writes in *Memoirs of a Woman of Pleasure* (NY: G. P. Putnam's Sons, 1963) that Louisa and a man engage in "turtle-billing kisses, and the poignant painless love-bites" (131). What is important to note here is that the scratching and biting is basically painless. When we are aroused, the line between pain and pleasure becomes blurred, especially with the nerve endings of the skin. So one must scrape the fingernails along the back with more pressure in order to cause discomfort when we are aroused. But the kind of biting and scratching depicted on TV, in films and in books—where blood flows—goes beyond what can cause pain/pleasure for most people.

11. See the previous chapter about role playing. Such depictions are the result of two things. First, they are a carry-over from the days[a] when males thought they were superior and in control—when a man "took" a woman. (See the previous chapter about role playing.) It was thought that women didn't like sex[b] and had to be overpowered or that they liked what is now called "date rape" or "acquaintance rape." It was felt that women were the "weaker sex" and liked men "to take charge." And in sexual relations, as in all other relationships (political, economic, social, etc.), the strong dominate the weak (or think they do).

Second, many recent depictions of sexual activity are a reaction to the first idea. At some point it was decided that women should be treated and depicted just like men. Women don't dislike sex; they love it. If women are just like men, then they too must be aggressive; they must want to dominate; they must like their pleasure mixed with pain.

One of the great disappointments of the various social movements of the 1960s is that those who achieved some measure of liberation and equality—blacks and women, for example—have not used the opportunity to bring about fundamental changes. Women are now afforded the opportunity to develop heart disease sooner by working in stress-filled, male-dominated occupations. Blacks can now appear in toilet-bowl-cleaner advertisements and "star" in mindless situation comedies. Liberation and equality means only, unfortunately, the freedom to do the same things that have always been done. It's true that some important changes have taken place (some men, for example, now take a larger and more active role in raising children), but most of the achievements of the 60s have been frittered away.[c]

Something similar is happening in Eastern Europe and the former Soviet Union. While they were oppressed, we saw only glimpses of their contemporary music, literature, and drama; it seemed that each Eastern European had a secret creative life. Now that they have thrown off many of the shackles of Communism, we do not see a burst of creative activity as had been hoped. Instead there has been an explosion of interest in scandal-sheets, pornography, and astrology. What many forget is that true freedom is the freedom to be stupid, brutal, apathetic, and greedy as well as intelligent, caring, concerned and generous. True freedom is accompanied by responsibility. The unfree are not responsible, since they are not free to choose or do. The free may be greedy, but they must bear the consequences of their greed. Excuse me: I find that I have unintentionally veered into demagoguery ("the outward sign of the populist's inner grace," says Gore Vidal).[d]

Currently there seems to be another reaction taking place. Whereas for centuries men were depicted as (and, it must be admitted, generally were) aggressive and dominant, their "new-age" brothers are sensitive, concerned, sympathetic, and sharing. Action and reaction—always the pudendulum swings too widely. Of course, some men are caring individuals. But many are aggressive dolts. Many are sensitive to the needs of their lovers, but many are uncaring oafs. Some are tender and some are brutal. The same is true of women. Some are gentle and some are cruel. Some are intelligent and some are mindless bimbos. Some women are leaders and some are sheep. Avoid stereotypes and simplistic rationalizations.

12. It is quite possible that your "friends" are questioning your intention to begin Swell-Wimp. They may say that it sounds crazy. Well, tell them that teasers at the beginning of the evening news shows are crazy, and square headlights on automobiles are crazy, and nail-care franchises are crazy, and fuel-air explosives are crazy, and, well, again I have digressed.[e]

13. However, we are not without training in this area. We both took a sociology course as undergraduates and during our Swell-Wimp studies we have come face-to-face with society's problems first hand.

14. We have experimented (after all we are scientists) with aggressive (even violent) SexAct, but neither of us likes it personally.

15. Or as the narrator of Laurence Sterne's *Tristram Shandy* says, "so long as a man rides his HOBBY-HORSE peaceably and quietly along the King's highway, and neither compels you or me to get up behind him,—pray, Sir, what have either you or I to do with it?" (Indianapolis: The Odyssey Press, 1940, 13).

16. Emily Dickinson, living as she did without much experience of the world at large, was deluded at first about the size of the penis; she believed what little she had heard from others at school and thought that an erect penis was a gigantic thing. Imagine how Emily Dickinson's partner (a scrivener named Mac Flecknoe) felt after her comment (Poem 271):

> And would it feel as big—
> When I could take it in my hand—
> As hovering—seen—through fog—
>
> ....
>
> Swelled—like Horizons—in my vest—
> And I sneered—softly—"small"!

17. Willy-nilly; With one voice; Standing on one foot; To everyone, his [or her] own is beautiful; To use, not abuse.

18. You should probably avoid singing the blues, dirges, and laments.

19. C. Hugh Holman defines a double entendre as a "statement that is deliberately ambiguous, one of whose possible meanings is risqué or suggestive of some impropriety" (*A Handbook to Literature*, 3rd ed. (Indianapolis: Bobbs-Merrill, 1972). For example, the state motto of Wyoming: *cedant arma toqae*, means "let arms yield to the gown." Those who approved it probably thought it meant something like "let military power be subordinate to civil authority" and not "let men yield to women." The motto of New Mexico, *crescit eundo* means "it grows as it goes"!

20. For example, the old favorite:

> Y'all come.
> 'N' I'll come.
> We'll come together, yessiree!

Or to the tune of "Kiss Me, Once," you might sing "Spank me, once. 'N' spank me, twice. 'N' spank me, once again." Substitute your favorite verb.

21. She: You say blow job.
    He: I say fellatio.
    She: You say poontang.
    He: I say intercourse.
    Together: Let's call the whole thing off (not really).

22. He: I came nine times.
    She: You came eight.
    He: We were on time.
    She: No, you were late.
    He: Ah, yes. I remember it well.

23. Kiss, kiss, kiss my breasts.
    Make my nipples firm.
    Hug me,

Stroke me,
Lick me,
Kiss, me,
But, please don't mess my perm.

24. If you are really ambitious, you could sing Emily Dickinson's ode to multiple orgasms (Poem 598) to the tune of "The Battle Hymn of the Republic":

Three times—we parted—Breath—and I—
Three times—He would not go—
....
Three times—the Billows tossed me up—
Then caught me—like a Ball—
....
The Waves grew sleepy—Breath—did not—
The Winds—like Children—lulled—
Then Sunrise kissed my chrysalis—
And I stood up—and lived—

25. "Pessimistic Rumination in Popular Songs and News Magazines Predict Economic Recession via Decreased Consumer Optimism and Spending," *Journal of Economic Psychology*, 1991.

26. The original lyrics to this Irish folk tune were not the familiar "Danny Boy" lyrics.

27. The ancient Indians classified the sounds made during climax and compared them to various bird cries; they also warned against having mynahs and parrots near where you make love.

28. For more suggestions, see the entry for "Coitus" in *Grove's Dictionary of Music and Musicians* (NY: St. Martin's Press, 1955) and Euterpe Erato, "Sooterkin Songs," *Chambre Syndicale de les Grandes Horizontales Americaine*, 69:23–40.

29. If you are generally not a happy, smiling person, you might purchase *Kokigamii: The Intimate Art of the Little Paper Costume* by Heather Busch and Burton Silver (Berkeley, CA: Ten Speed Press, 1992). The book contains paper cutouts (origami) that are used to transform the penis into familiar creatures and objects (horse, fish, pig, dragon, steam engine, space shuttle, fire engine, dog). Included are scripts to be acted out. You will find it hard not to smile when you "make the doggie go bow-wow."

30. Even better would be repeated arousal and climax, but this is not possible for men. Although women can achieve orgasm many times, men can rarely ejaculate

more than twice in a short time. Of course, "macho" men would have us believe that they can "do it" all night long, but "it" must be something other than orgasm. C. F.

31. Incidentally, feathers are good for tickling and arousing because they raise goosebumps which expend energy. See Appendix A for more on goosebumps.

32. Unless one is very insecure. Also, although *dulce est desipare in loco* (it's good to relax and be silly), timing can be crucial; laughter can cause either partner to fail at the moment of climax.

33. See Michel Foucault, *Les Mots et les choses* (1966); reprinted as *The Order of Things: An Archaeology of the Human Sciences* (NY: Vintage Books, 1973), 343.

34. See, for example, *Overcoming Relationship Impasses: Ways to Initiate Change When Your Partner Won't Help* by Barry L. Duncan and Joseph W. Rock (NY: Plenum Publishing, 1991) and Norman Rush's 1991 National Book Award-winning study *Mating* (NY: A. A. Knopf, 1991).

35. Geoffery Chaucer uses this word frequently in *The Tales of Canterbury* spelling it variously as "queynte," "kent," and "queinte."

36. Forum Adviser: The Answers To Every Question You Ever Had About Sex, Penthouse Forum Magazine, 1977.

37. Or "spill a few fire drops of impatience" as the narrator of *Transparent Things* by Vladimir Nabokov ([NY: McGraw-Hill, 1972], 35) says.

38. Boccaccio warns that "to thwart the laws of Nature requires too much strength, especially as those who labour to do so, not only labour in vain, but to their own great harm" (*The Decameron*, 251).

39. Masters, Johnson and Kolodny refer to this point in males (at which ejaculation cannot be stopped) as "ejaculatory inevitability" (*On Sex and Human Loving* (Boston & Toronto: Little, Brown and Co., 1982), 71). They have no similar term for women.

40. It is best to choose carefully when, where and to whom you speak. [ed.]

41. With great noise. [jed]

Chapter 7

1. *Sexual Behavior in the Human Male*, 366.

2. *Sexual Behavior in the Human Female*, 365.

3. The advice in this chapter generally applies to those who cross dress, although we don't specifically discuss the topic.

Males wearing female garments is much more common than females wearing male garments. So many male comics (Milton Berle and Robin Williams from two different eras for example) wear female clothing for laughs that it seems to be a rite of passage. Most serious male actors at some point in their careers cross dress (for example, Cary Grant and Dustin Hoffman, again from different times). There is no way of knowing how many males secretly wear women's clothing, occasionally or frequently. It does seem that every male will do so publicly and eagerly, if the circumstances allow it. Rarely does an episode of one of the TV home-video shows not include at least one clip of a man dressed in female clothing, usually underwear. The conclusion to be drawn from all this is so obvious that I'll refrain from commenting. C. F.

4. Choosing appropriate garments is relatively easy compared to the subjects that Vatsyayana in *Kama Sutra* says should be studied. For example, women should study tattooing; coloring of the teeth, garments, hair, nails and bodies; applying perfumed ointments and perfumes to the body and hair; and gymnastics.

5. It has been suggested that some of our advice in this chapter goes a bit far. However, Alex Comfort in *The New Joy of Sex* (NY: Crown Publishers, 1991) refers to a man who did just this (wore diving equipment during sex) and further required that rubber sheets be used on the bed! Nothing we suggest could be more outrageous than what people already do. Some people seem to live according to the principle of *credo quia absurdum est* (I believe because it is absurd). When it comes to SexAct even the absurd is believable.

6. However, winter footwear, designed to keep your feet warm, is not so good, because it is cumbersome and few people need to lose weight in their feet.

7. You must be very careful with plastic bags. Don't put them over your head; you may suffocate. Do not wear them for long periods of time; all of the body's parts need to "breathe." Don't let children play with them. Dispose of them properly so that children, animals and your partner won't be injured. They are such good suffocators, that they are recommended as a second line of defense against failed suicide in Derek Humphry's book, *Final Exit* (Eugene, Oregon: The Hemlock Society, 1991).

8. Fewer people would be injured and killed if the following message were printed INSIDE all plastic bags: "If you can read this you are endangering your life! Remove your head from this bag immediately!" Along with the printed message there should be a picture of a big, hairy, ugly monster-face to frighten children.

9. However, see Chapter 10 about SexEx in the cold to increase calorie consumption.

10. To prevent injuries, avoid caps and hats from which things dangle, such as tassels, balls, fishing licenses and lures, and so on.

11. However, some people find it more exciting when it is difficult or complicated to remove footwear.

12. *Kama Sutra*, Chapter 3 of Part 1, and Chapter 2 of Part 2. The word shampoo is derived from a Hindi word for "massage."

13. Primitive is not used pejoratively here. It is not synonymous with barbaric and refers to many societies. Maybe simple or uncomplex would be a better term. There are a number of contemporary societies that are quite sophisticated, and thus not primitive, but they are barbaric. Jean Auel in the Earth's Children series of books has convincingly shown that prehistoric peoples were not socially or culturally unsophisticated. Nor were they sexually primitive or barbaric: Ayla and Jondalar are caring, sensitive, sophisticated lovers and can serve as paradigms for us today.

14. Of course, there is also the situation where a dying person wants to look good in order to meet his or her maker.

15. The lover Berenice, famous for her beautiful hair, was immortalized by having a constellation named for her. And Belinda, in Alexander Pope's Rape of the Lock is given the same honor. See also two notes forward.

16. Too much should not be made of this analogy though. Samson was a Nazarene, one especially dedicated to God; as such he did not drink wine, go near dead bodies or cut his hair.

17. And, of course, there are Chaucer's wonderful lines in "The Miller's Tale" (ll. 3732–3741):

> And at the wyndow out she putte her hole
> And Absolon, hym fil no bet ne wers,
> But with his mouth he kiste hir naked ers
> Ful savourly, er he were war of this.
> Abak he stirte, and thoughte it amys,
> For wel he wiste a womman hath no berd.
> He felt a thyng al rough and long yherd
> And sayde, "Fy! allas! what have I do?"
> "Tehee!" quode she, and clapte the wyndow to
> And Absolon gooth forth a sory pas.

18. See two notes back.

19. Authors also use the facial hair of men as symbols too. A neat trimmed beard or mustache can indicate a fastidious character while a long wild beard can indicate an insane or liberated personality.

20. Occasionally, an author will remark on the hair on a woman's arms (T. S. Eliot's "The Love Song of J. Alfred Prufrock") or her upper lip or chin (Vladimir Nabokov).

21. Of course, *de omni re scibili et quibusdom aliis*: we know many things, but we haven't read every piece of literature written in the last twenty-five years.

22. As evidenced by Timbuk 3's "Hairstyles" and Christine Lavin's "I Love Bald-Headed Men" rising to eighth and fourth on the pop-music charts.

23. Additionally, your hair choice can have tremendous political and cultural significance. Professor Kennell Jackson, a member of the history department, taught a course titled "Black Hair as Culture and History" during the 1992 Spring semester at Stanford University.

24. Very short hair with shaved areas is currently popular with males. But our female study participants complained that short hair made some activities, especially cunnilingus, very uncomfortable for them.

25. Queen Elizabeth established it as acceptable and Sinead O'Connor has made it chic.

26. I understand this is now called "going commando," but I don't know why. When I was young it was called "skivvies-less".

27. Of course, some men regularly shave their penis so that the hairs do not become entangled in a condom—a most unpleasant experience.

28. Vatsyayana in *Kama Sutra* says that a man should get his head and face shaved every four days and other parts of his body every five or ten days.

29. Interestingly, males shaving their armpits does not seem to be very stimulating, although some men who work in suits and ties do this to reduce the amount of perspiration retained there.

30. In general, male body hair is coarser than female body hair, probably because of hormones. A recent cover of *Discover* magazine showed a picture of a "cave woman" with shaved legs. God knows how the photo survived, but it clearly demonstrates that our modern attitude toward women shaving their legs had its roots in prehistory.

31. Noni Hazlehurst played Nora, an attractive contemporary (1970s) woman in her thirties, with hairy armpits in the 1982 Australian film *Monkey Grip* based on Helen Garner's novel (Melbourne: McPhee Gribble, 1977). In Vladimir Nabokov's *Glory* (trans. Dimitri Nabokov [NY: McGraw-Hill, 1971] 147), written in 1932, the narrator tells us that Sonia (about 20 years old) "put her bare arms behind her head, exposing her lovely armpits which she had recently started to shave and which were now shaded as if with a pencil...."

32. Alex Comfort says that armpit hair, "Should on no account be shaved" (66) although he says a woman's can be cut in a hot climate without plumbing (49). He prefers natural odors and does not like deodorants. He makes no distinction in this section between male and female armpit hair. We do not take such an absolutist position; to shave or not is your choice; there are advantages and disadvantages to both.

33. In the past the armpit was admired much more than today. The Arabs even placed it in the firmament: the name of the star Betelgeuse in the constellation Orion means "armpit."

34. Notice for example, provincial Franz's reaction to sophisticated city-dwelling Martha ("he was stunned to observe that her armpits were as smooth and white as a statue's") in Nabokov's *King. Queen, Knave* (NY: McGraw-Hill, 1968, 83). And this from Émile Zola's *Nana* (trans. George Holden [Baltimore; Penguin Books, 1972]) set in nineteenth-century France: "This was Venus rising from the waves, with no veil save her tresses. And when Nana raised her arms, the golden hairs in her arm-pits could be seen in the glare of the footlights" (44). Or this from Vladimir Nabokov's *Ada or Ardor* (NY: McGraw-Hill, 1960): "[Lucette]…readjusting her green helmet, with touchingly graceful movements of her raised wings, and touchingly flashing the russet feathering of her armpits" (479).

35. Unless it is small and covered by several layers of clothing as is the case with buttocks, breast and genitalia painting, which many people find very stimulating. (It is said that the 14th President of the United States was an advocate of nipple and penis piercing. The suits that were worn in the nineteenth century hid them from view, but he knew and that's what's important.) Still, buttock, breast and genitalia painting is likely to smear and fade because of the high humidity in these areas.

36. SoHo artist Lesley Dill applies a white base to naked models' bodies, writes Emily Dickinson's poems on them, poses them and photographs them. You might expect, since this "art form" combines Dickinson and nakedness, that we would approve but we don't. Although Dill rightly perceives that Dickinson's poetry is sensual, even erotic, putting the poems on naked bodies distracts from the poetry and the white base abstracts the bodies so as to deny their inherent sensuality. Thus, each part is diminished and the sum of the parts is not greater than the whole.

37. And good merkins are really expensive.

38. See Aldo Busi, *The Standard Life of a Temporary Pantyhose Salesman* (Italy, 1985; Britain, 1989).

39. A female leg that has not been shaved in four weeks is most arousing, but one that has not been shaved in four days is a nasty thing. P. B.

The same might be said of a man's beard. C. F.

40. Great things are the result of small causes.

41. As an experiment, I attempted to live naked for two weeks (at home and at the lab); I kept the house and lab at 63 degrees and maintained my normal diet and activities. After three days I gave up; I just couldn't get used to the cold. I lost 3.9 pounds, but since I was shivering frequently I can't state to what degree goosebumps (nearly continuous) contributed to my weight loss. How do nudists do it?

42. She was a beauty "touched with fraise in four places, a symmetrical queen of hearts" (Nabokov, *Ada*, 375).

43. Actually, bald-headed people radiate more heat through their heads than do people with full heads of hair. Thus, allowing your hair to grow will increase your energy expenditure if your engage in SexEx in a warm location because the body will have to work harder to cool itself. C. F.

44. Shaving all of your body hair (head and pubic region included) will decrease your weight from a few ounces to several pounds depending upon how large your body is, how hairy you are, and how long your hair has been allowed to grow. But since this has nothing to do with body fat and being overweight, it should not be thought of as weight reduction.

45. *Non mihi, non tibi, sed nobis.* [ed.]

46. In 1861 British naturalist Henry Walter Bates proposed that a nontoxic species, to increase the odds against being eaten, could evolve to look just like a toxic one. In the 1890s the British evolutionary biologist E. B. Poulton claimed that the nontoxic Viceroy butterfly, which looks like the toxic Monarch butterfly, was an example of Bates' evolutionary theory (the non-toxic species evolves to look like the toxic species. We now know that both butterflies taste bad.) Similarly, there was a time when a woman might dress like a slut in order to look easy and thus pick up guys more easily. Now, she might dress that way in order to keep men away because she looks like someone who might have AIDS. P. B.

Indeed! C. F.

47. I have an idea for a piece of clothing that I think would be very popular. I don't have the means to produce it myself, and the manufacturers to which I wrote didn't even respond, so I'd like to share it with you. Basically, the garment is a pair of pants or shorts with open sides. First, imagine opening the legs of a pair of jeans by cutting the two outside seams. Now imagine rejoining them using four (or more) straps—one at the cuff, knee, thigh and hip—leaving a gap of one-half to one inch. So, instead of being joined tightly and continuously from cuff to hip, the outside seams are joined loosely and at four points. Through the gap one could see a portion of the wearer's hips, legs, socks and underwear (if he or she was wearing underwear). This basic

design could be used for dozens of kinds of apparel—polyester walking shorts, jeans, work-out shorts, dress trousers, stirrup-pants and so on. Now imagine that the straps are not anchored by stitching but by buttons, snaps or Velcro which can be easily and quickly undone. One could don the item by opening two attachments at the hips instead of a button or snap and zipper in the front. The item could be loose-fitting or skin-tight. This would be a very sexy garment, affording just a glimpse of flesh, but a glimpse where we usually don't see bare body. Clothing for men and women could be made this way, revealing a masculine hairy leg and hip or a smooth female leg and hip. Visualize going to the disco in beautiful designer jeans with a strip of flesh showing from hip to ankle, revealing just a glimpse of bikini underwear (or no underwear at all). What could be seen through the gap is actually much less than a low-cut or high-hemmed dress shows, but it would reveal the body in a new way. It would also make panties and shorts part of the visual ensemble. This is a guaranteed hot-selling item. And IT'S MINE. If someone reading this would be interested in making a deal to manufacture these items of clothing, he or she can contact me through my publisher and make arrangements for royalties or outright purchase of the design (or whatever is done in the garment industry). P. B.

48. One day President Calvin Coolidge's wife exclaimed to him about a rooster's ability to mate many times in a single day. He replied it was true, but the rooster was not stuck with only one hen. The Coolidge Effect is the tendency of a sexually-satiated individual to be turned on by a new partner. P. B.

Either partner can be affected by the Coolidge Effect—hens as well as roosters. C. F.

Chapter 8

1. This is contrary to the spirit of Swell-Wimp—an easy, INEXPENSIVE, and pleasurable method of losing weight and maintaining fitness through sexual activity.

2. There is little good sex in prison.

3. Vatsyayana in Part 1, Chapter 3 of *Kama Sutra* says that one of the subjects that women should study is gymnastics. We don't think this is necessary, although it can be helpful.

4. However, too much control can be a problem also. Sam Izdat in "The Sad End of Frau Zwei Hummerbuns' Marriage," *Coprolites*, November 1923, 65–69 relates the consequences of overdeveloping muscle control. Frau Hummerbuns would flex her buttock muscles alternately when she went to bed and she and her husband were

cuddled like spoons (lying on their sides with his belly against her back, his penis between her thighs). The buttock flexing was a little game: she'd say she was exercising and it would usually cause him to get an erection. Eventually, she was able to tighten and relax her muscles so quickly that her buttocks would vibrate, producing a humming noise. Her husband was not pleased by this development and eventually he divorced her because she began to make her buttocks hum in public.

5. "The Pain Perplex," *The New Yorker*, 21 Sept. 1998, 88.

6. "Low-Back Pain," *Scientific American*, August 1998, 52.

7. It is unfortunate that the medical establishment has not made this fact public. Why don't physicians[a] tell us about this? Is it because back injury is a very profitable ailment? Once they have determined that a patient's back problems are not due to something severe, such as a fracture, they should tell their patients to go easy on SexAct for a while and explain the exercises that they can do to strengthen their backs.

8. "Low-Back Pain," 49.

9. Some might argue that there were fewer back problems because they engaged in SexAct less frequently and thus didn't injured themselves as often. It is possible to gather data from diaries, letters, memoirs and such and extrapolate from the few to the general, but this has not been done yet. Studies of the Puritans, whom we think of as morally straight-laced and even sexually repressed, indicate that they were no less sexually active in private than we are (indeed they were less public about it). And studies of Victorian England come to the same conclusion. Thus, the lower incidence of back problems during these times is probably due, not to less frequent SexAct, but to more physical labor which made their backs stronger which prevented injuries during sexual climax. Of course, it is difficult to accurately determine how common back problems were in past times.

10. Harvey L. and Jean S. Gochros in *The Sexually Oppressed* (NY: Associated Press, 1977) say "As much as 80 percent of backaches are due to muscle fatigue rather than slipped discs or arthritis" (70).

11. "Low-Back Pain," 52.

12. When your back gets really strong, place objects in a backpack and wear it while exercising.

13. From behind. [ed.]

14. Only humans, primates, and elephants have a single set of breasts on the "chest." Other species have multiple pairs elsewhere.

15. In the 18th century, breasts were colloquially called bubbies; today they are called boobies.

16. The average breast size in Britain today is 36-B. We can find no data for the United States, but the size should be about the same. Occasionally, only one breast will grow to adult size before the other does; usually the other catches up. It is normal for one of an adult woman's breasts to be a cup-size larger than the other.

17. Dr. Wayne Kotter says that it's not "The bigger they are, the harder they fall," [b] but "The bigger they are, the more likely they're fake."

18. Did you know that in Wyoming about three-quarters of a mile south of Peak 49 there is a twin peak named Maidenform Peak (elevation 11,137)?

19. In *Futz*, the 1967 play by Rochelle Owens, Farmer Futz is in love with his sow, Amanda. The pig may be imaginary, but he asks, "How many tits does *your* wife have?...Mine has twelve"! David Reuben, *Everything You Always Wanted to Know About Sex* reports that approximately one woman in two hundred has three or more nipples; however, it is extremely rare for a woman to have an extra breast.

20. We do not recommend or approve of breast enlargement surgery. Breast reduction surgery is sometimes warranted.

21. Vatsyayana classifies women into three kinds—Mrigi (deer), Vadawa (mare) and Hastini (elephant)—according to the depth of her "yoni" (vagina), but he is referring to the extremely small or large woman. He also gives directions for using fruits and roots for contracting the yoni of an Elephant woman and enlarging the yoni of a Deer woman. Neither procedure results in useful, permanent changes.

The male ego is a fragile (read juvenile) thing; many men believe their penis is larger than normal and that they are a special treat for women (if she can take it!). The facts are that (1) an adult woman's vagina is tremendously elastic and can accommodate a penis of almost any size, (2) most men have (surprise) average-sized penises, and (3) even a smaller-than-average penis can provide a woman with pleasure because it is the exterior rubbing against the clitoris that is important. It cannot be denied that the presence and movement of the penis in the vagina provides pleasure for most women, but is not the primary source (contrary to that ridiculous old man's theory of the vaginal orgasm). C. F.

22. in the walls of the vagina leads to moisture seeping across

23. However, the presence of vaginal lubrication does not automatically mean the woman is ready for intercourse. C. F.

24. Did you know that "hae" in Cantonese means "yes," but with a change of pitch it means pudendum, a woman's external genital organs, the vulva? Pudendum is derived from the Latin for "to be ashamed." Pudenda (plural) refers to the external sex organs of both sexes.

25. The word "clitoris" is derived from the Greek, meaning "key." It is also called "penis Muliebris," meaning "penis of woman."

26. Admittedly, this is an advanced technique that few women are willing to devote the time to developing. Still, it shows how much control women have compared to men. C. F.

27. See Chapter 5.

28. Do not TOTALLY release these muscles or you will go pee-pee or poo-poo.

29. There is also a psychological pleasure resulting from the knowledge that you have control of your sexual apparatus in a way and to a degree that your male partner does not. But as we mentioned before, sadness may also result. C. F.

30. Even Vatsyayana recognized that there are short-timed, moderate-timed and long-timed women.

31. See Karen Wright, "Evolution of the Big O.," *Discover*, June 1992, 53–58.

32. Only 30% of the women in Shere Hite's study could regularly achieve orgasm from intercourse without more direct manual clitoral stimulation being provided. Yet, about one third of women claim to fake orgasms because the pressure is so great that they should. Hite refers to sexual intercourse as the Rube Goldberg method of female sexual fulfillment.

33. In general, a man's penis appears shorter to him than to others because of the viewing angle when he looks down at it.

34. Vatsyayana in Part 2, Chapter 1 of *Kama Sutra* classifies men according to the size of their penises: hare, bull and horse. In Part 3, Chapter 2, he explains how to enlarge the penis by rubbing it with the bristles of certain insects and oil. However, this is an unpleasant experience and does not result in a useful, permanent enlargement.

35. Diane Kelly, in a paper titled "Axial Orthogonal Fiber Reinforcement in the Penis of the Nine-Banded Armadillo," showed that the cylinder of the penis is not surrounded by longitudinal or circumferential fibers but by axial orthogonal fibers (see Mary Roach, "Intimate Engineering," *Discover*, Feb. 1999). The significance of this is that until very recently it was believed that all penises had helical reinforcing fibers. Apparently, until Ms. Kelly, no "scientist" was sufficiently curious to take a close look. Most scientists are no smarter, no more curious or skeptical than the average citizen (what, in fact, is a "scientist"?). Scientific progress is hampered by the "everybody knows" syndrome. Kelly also says that little is actually known about the biomechanics of ejaculation. We should not unquestioningly accept information (scientific, economic, historic, etc.) just because the writer or speaker has advanced degrees.

36. Note deleted. [ed.]

37. However, an erection is so fragile that a sudden noise, a critical word or a disapproving look can bring about catastasis. The penis remains limp for twenty to sixty minutes after ejaculation, but men who haven't had sex in a long time or are intensely stimulated may recuperate in five minutes. Many men lie about how often they do it and how fast they recuperate because of societal pressures: peers expect it; movies and books depict it. The penis sometimes remains erect for five minutes or so after orgasm; we don't know why this happens, but it is normal.

38. Paintings on ancient Greek vases show that the Athenians used wreaths for the purpose of strengthening the penis. See Gary Wills, "Athena's Magic," *The New York Review of Books,* December 17, 1992, 50.

39. Glazed doughnuts are very high in calories so don't use one every time you do this exercise unless your partner is underweight.

40. Alex Comfort in *The New Joy of Sex* (NY: Crown Publishers, 1991) claims that the amount of fluid ejaculated can be increased by masturbating almost to orgasm an hour before sex.

41. In men between 20 and 40, the prostate can become inflamed and cause feelings of fullness and pain in the perineum between the testicles and the anus. After 40, 60% of men experience some enlargement of the prostate which can block the urethra. See Chapter 14 for more information.

42. Thus, dressing very warmly to sweat and lose weight can also reduce potency. Studies have shown that male potency goes down during the summer months, especially among males who wear tight pants and spend much time in the heat. However, this cannot serve as birth control. Nor can cooling the testicles by placing them in a cold bath (which some primitive peoples do). The reduction in potency is not complete. On the other hand, if you and your partner are trying to conceive, you can increase your chances by not decreasing potency by wearing tight clothing which will give you a hot crotch.

43. Male kangaroos fight by leaning back upon their tails and using their clawed, hind feet to rip at their opponents abdomen. When they fight their testicles are drawn completely into the abdominal cavity for protection. This is true of other animals as well. Is it possible that men once fought by jumping up and clawing at their enemy's abdomens with their toe nails? C. F.

44. ! C. F.

45. We mean increase in the positive sense. Of course, hitting them with a hammer will cause enlargement and several medical conditions will produce swelling.

46. Fellatio is oral stimulation of the penis; that is, stimulating the penis with the lips, teeth and tongue; ejaculation may or may not result; the penis may or may not be taken into the mouth. The word is derived from the Latin for "suck." Cunnilingus is oral stimulation of the clitoris or vulva with the lips, teeth and tongue. It is derived from the Latin for "he who licks the vulva." Needless to say, you must be very careful when using your teeth during fellatio and cunnilingus. David Reuben in *Everything You Always Wanted to Know About Sex* (NY: Bantam Books, 1969) claims that 70% to 80% of Americans engage in fellatio and cunnilingus.

47. There was a woman on a recent television video show (America's or World's or Universe's funniest or something) who could independently raise either side, the front, middle and back of her tongue and with such speed as to simulate waves, smiley faces and so on. I wish I had had the VCR on at that time. Her ability to control her tongue deserves study; I, personally, would like to know how she does it.

48. For more information see Bill Bryson, *The Mother Tongue* (NY: William Morrow, 1990).

49. Although almost universally practiced by all peoples of all times, oral sex has often been characterized as indecent. Vatsyayana refers to fellatio and cunnilingus as Auparishtaka or mouth congress—activities engaged in primarily by eunuchs, unchaste and wanton women, attendants, serving maids and women of the harem (with each other). What we today call "69"—when a man and woman lie face to feet and perform mutual oral stimulation—he called (we can't imagine why) "congress of the crow." Incidentally, there is no such thing as a "blow-job." It's simply impossible to cause an orgasm by blowing on the sex organs. Its existence is a myth perpetuated for untold years by adolescent males and recently by journalists covering the Clinton-Lewinsky affair. Although much has been written about fellatio, hum-jobs, sucking-off, and giving head, we can find nothing about "blow-job" or "getting blown" in any of the academic literature. Neither of us has experienced it.

50. We mean here the nose in the middle of the man's face through which he breathes, and not the penis which is frequently euphemistically referred to as the nose. See, for example, *The Life and Opinions of Tristram Shandy* by Laurence Sterne (1759–1767).

51. For more information see William Cullen, *Nosology* (NY: Alan Sokal Imprints, 1991).

52. Interestingly, the same thing happens when we become angry, another psycho-emotional state.

53. However, we would be interested in hearing from anyone who can demonstrate/document the use of nostril flaring as a pleasurable activity during SexAct.

Since the use of any muscle burns up calories, this activity could conceivably become another energy-expending Swell-Wimp activity.

54. Although a firm, persistent erection is desirable, Priapism is not. This is a condition in which a man has an intense, prolonged erection; it just doesn't go down. The pain is excruciating and it may last for weeks. Surgery seems to be the only treatment if the condition does not cure itself. The term is derived from Priapus, the Greco-Roman god of procreation who was usually depicted as having a huge erect penis. Paradoxically, in Petronius' *Satirycon*, Encolpius incurs the wrath of Priapus and his punishment is impotence. Thus, the term priapism is illogical. In any case Priapus translates into modern English as "Richard." The modern followers of Priapus engage in Richardic rites.

55. As we've pointed out before, SexEx burns up from 80 to 480 calories per hour. So you would have to engage in SexEx for one to two hours to equal the number of calories expended during twenty minutes of aerobic exercise. But as we've asked before—wouldn't you rather?

56. Too much exercise is not good. [ed.]

57. There are no easy solutions to life's complicated problems. At the turn of the century, Sherlock Holmes would determine whether a man was a libertine or a pillar of the community based on his handwriting! We all know that's impossible (even if Holmes wasn't fictional). But just a few years ago in 1991 Marie Bernard published *Sexual Deviations as Seen in Handwriting* (Genf: Ariston, 1994). Who bought her book? Does the fact that she calls herself a "graphologist," make readers think that what she claims to do is scientific? There is no easy way to determine whether a person is of good character. You should not be misled by such "pseudo-scientific" books. Be moderate and be skeptical.

Chapter 9

1. Or, as Emily Dickinson says in Poem 271, "to drop a life/ Into the purple well."

2. If you have been engaging in sex primarily for pleasure and are not entirely clear about the procreative aspects, you should read one or more of the following: *The Golden Book of Making Babies* (1945), "Night-Sea Journey" by John Barth in *Lost in the Funhouse* (NY: Bantam Books, 1963), or *My Child Is a Mother* (San Antonia: Corona Publishing, 1992) by Mary Stephensen. Of course, you can consult a physician (obstetrician, gynecologist, pederast, or general practitioner) for information.

3. Research now indicates that the egg is not passive, but calls the sperm via chemical signals and captures the sperm which are actually trying to escape. See David H. Freedman, "The Aggressive Egg," *Discover*, June 1992, 61–65. C. F.

4. You might enjoy reading Sylvia Plath's "Metaphors." The first line says, "I'm a riddle in nine syllables" and the poem contains nine lines of nine syllables enumerating a number of metaphors for "pregnant." See also the section "A Flower in Your Apron" later in the chapter.

5. Be sure to read "Take Precautions" in Chapter 13.

6. *On Sex and Human Loving* (Boston & Toronto: Little, Brown and Co., 1982), 153.

7. Of course, some of the pregnancies are welcomed and some of the mothers and babies go on to lead happy productive lives. But it is almost certain that the statistics reflect more unhappiness than happiness.

8. Or "dupe procreation" as Nabokov says in *Ada or Ardor* (NY: McGraw-Hill, 1960), 15.

9. For a thorough discussion of the issue, see Joseph and Pamela Andrews, *Chastity: Two Views* (Berlin: Prignitz and Scroderus, 1969).

10. A long footnote castigating the Catholic Church for its blindness to the problem of overpopulation and, therefore, its criminal advocacy of depletion of the earth's resources has been deleted. [ted]

11. Everything You Wanted to Know About Sex But Were Afraid to Ask (NY: Bantam Books, 1969).

12. Condoms made from natural materials, an alternative for men who are allergic to latex condoms, offer no protection against AIDS.

13. W. V. Harris, "Old Wives' Tales," *The New York Review of Books*, 18 November 1993, 52–54.

14. "Sole sura metoda por decevor natura, est por un strong-guy de contino-contino-contino jusque le plesir brimz; et lors, a lultima instanta, svitchera a l'altra gropa; ma perquoi una femme ardora andor ponderosa ne se retorna kvik enof, la transita e facilitata per positio torvago." (from *On Contraceptive Devices* quoted in *Chastity: Two Views*, 156)

15. See also *The Cambridge Companion to Buggery* (NY: Cambridge University Press, 1979) and Jonathan Goldberg, *Sodometries* (Stanford, CA: Stanford Univ. Press, 1992).

16. Those of you who have not engaged in sexual activity (because of extreme obesity or whatever) for a long time (twenty-five years or more) should note that the birth control pill is meant to be regularly ingested by the female and not used to plug the penis.

17. They're about $4.00 per package cheaper if you order via the Internet, but you have to purchase at least a three-month supply—impossible for many low-income women.

18. I certainly agree with Dr. Flanders. Further, of the cost of prescription drugs what portion goes to pharmacies? And what do they do for their cut? They claim they check for adverse drug interactions, blah, blah, blah. The pharmacy where my mother gets her pills doesn't even own a computer and sends her hand-written bills! When I get my Dilantin prescription filled, I have to wait 20 minutes while the pharmacist takes pills from a big bottle and puts them into a little bottle and adds a label. This, it seems to me, constitutes 80% of what pharmacists do. Imagine going to the grocery store and paying someone for taking six rolls of toilet paper out of a big box and putting them in a smaller box. And, birth-control pills are pre-packaged, so the pharmacist doesn't even have to transfer pills from one bottle to another![a]

19. And surely not simultaneously.

20. Unfortunately, sometimes the tubes rejoin.

21. For a contrary view see Alexas Mardian, *The Most Unkindest Cuts of All* (NY: Mohel Books, 1989).

22. Unfortunately, sometimes the tubes rejoin.

23. Thus, the interest in and development of so many sexual positions (there are hundreds). Most were designed to enable the female to climax but prevent male climax by limiting the movement of the penis.

24. For a discussion of a Chinese method of avoiding pregnancy, see Bernard Boorsicot's *Shi Pei Pu: Pleasure Without Fear* (New York: Melpomene Books, 1992).

25. *The Hite Report* (NY: Macmillan; London: Collier Macmillan, 1976), 140.

26. Alexander Pope tells us that "Time was, a sober Englishman wou'd knock/ His servants up, and rise by five a clock" (*First Epistle of the Second Book of Horace Imitated*, ll. 161–162). Quite a feat, but in modern England birth control measures and the demise of the brutal, de-humanizing master-servant system have enabled women to choose when they will become pregnant.

27. This is probably (at least possibly) due to the fact that Western society has been male-dominated. If testicular cancer was as common as breast cancer, surgeons would have a different attitude about cutting off body parts. And if males became pregnant, there would be fewer Caesarean sections in the United States (of which it is estimated that 50,000 are unnecessary). C. F.

28. It doesn't matter which particular flower you have in mind—chrysanthemum, Hairy Alpine Rose, Daffodil, Pudendron, Lily—they're all beautiful.

29. The use of "apron" should not be taken as sexist. In the context of the story it does refer to a household apron. But today women wear many aprons—chef's, welder's, carpenter's, X-Ray technician's and so on—which are not symbols of subordination, but equality. P. B.

30. You don't want to experience the scare that Dickinson writes about in Poem 693:

> Wherefore so late—I murmured—
> My need of thee—be done—
> ....
> My Period begin [please]

31. I have been accused of being a bleeding-heart liberal. But I have also been called a mouthpiece for the right. Over just the last two years the following negative epithets have been hurled at me: extremist, naive, reactionary, feminist, sodomite, narrow-minded, poofter, poor scholar, secular humanist, ill-informed, apologist for this or that ism, lackey, anti-family, fool, humorless, hooligan, opportunist, bad writer, counter-revolutionary, money-grubbing capitalist, catamite, inept, pidgeon-toed, chauvinist, friggin' home-wrecker who better stay away from my wife, post-modernist, overweight, clueless, and politically-correct. Clearly those who attack me haven't taken the time to ponder my positions, which are complex and nuanced. Since I have been attacked by all sides, I tend to ignore criticism as uninformed passion.

Chapter 10

1. And psychological stamina. Further, women have better sight, hearing and sense of smell; they have better language skills, cooperative-working skills and holistic thinking skills; and they are better at long-term planning and implementation. See Helen Fisher, *The First Sex* (NY: Random House, 1999). C. F.

2. Apparently, this position was named by the Polynesians in reference to the manner in which the European missionaries performed intercourse. For more on the clash of cultural attitudes about sex, see *Pilgrim Path: The First Company of Women Missionaries to Hawaii* by Mary Zwiep (University of Wisconsin Press, 1992). Alex Comfort in *The New Joy of Sex* also calls it the matrimonial position and says that it is "uniquely satisfying." He points out that it is the ideal quick-orgasm position for both sexes and that it is easy to move to other positions from it. However, it may not be a good position if the man is overweight[a] or if the woman is pregnant.

Bonobos, also known as pygmy chimpanzees, are smaller and more delicate in build than chimpanzees. They are the only mammal, other than humans, that copulate face-to-face. Sexually they are more like humans than any other species: the female's clitoris and sexual swellings are oriented far forward like a human female's. They separate sex from reproduction, treating it as a pleasurable activity. They also engage in homosexual practices: females rub their genitals together and young males engage in fellatio. Bonobos engage in SexAct a lot, especially in stressful situations to relieve the anxiety and to bind the group together (Meredith F. Small, "What's Love Got to Do With It?" *Discover*, June 1992, 48–49).

3. In *The Perfect Fit: How to Achieve Mutual Fulfillment and Monogamous Passion Through the New Intercourse* (NY: Donald Fine, 1992), Edward Eichel and Philip Nobile describe the Coital Alignment Technique (CAT). This is nothing more than a modified missionary position with gentle tilting instead of pushing. CAT probably results in less energy expenditure, and as for pleasure, different strokes for different folks.

4. A variant form of "knock." [ed.]

5. Generally, we use "bed" in describing many of the techniques, but you may use any surface you like: cot, table, boat dock, ping pong table, pickup truck bed, car roof, kitchen counter, or whatever. You can perform SexAct wherever you please; if you and your partner like it and it gives you pleasure (or at least doesn't cause you pain) and it doesn't get you in trouble (where is the car located when you climb upon the roof?), then go ahead. Alex Comfort points out that some follies like engaging in some type of sexual activity in a public restaurant or appearing in public with only an overcoat over your naked body can be fun and stimulating. We agree. When I (P. B.) was an intern (in the "Lifestyles" division of the *Scranton Times* during my senior year of college), another intern and I "had sex" on the roof of the building during the daytime. It was certainly thrilling, but if we had been caught, our internships would have ended and possibly we would have been dismissed from college. So be careful.

6. *The New Joy of Sex*, 199 has a good illustration of this position under the heading "Inversion." Comfort calls "inversion" those positions in which the male's or female's head hangs down, as off the edge of the bed. We can verify his assertion that the buildup of pressure in the veins of the face and neck in this position during orgasm can give startling results—usually, but not always, enhancing the orgasm.

7. Vatsyayana says that women who have recently given birth, women who are menstruating and fat women should not "act the part of a man"—that is, take the top position (Chapter 8, *Kama Sutra*). However, the reverse missionary position (the woman on top) is very good for her because she has greater control of her movements

than when she is pinned in a position of submission by her partner (missionary position). She can manipulate her pelvic region so as to maximize clitoral stimulation; in fact, this is the position in which a woman is most likely to achieve orgasm through intercourse alone. C. F.

8. I'm told that Elizabeth Ard's book *Arms Control Development* (NY: Saurian Books, 1973) contains a thorough discussion of developing the arms rather than the entire upper body. P. B.

9. Either lower partner can help support the upper partner. Although, in general, men are stronger in the upper body than women, many men are very weak in this region.

10. Only one of our test subjects found this reverse clinging-dog position pleasurable and none of the females did.

11. Positions in which the female entirely supports the weight of the male are not unknown, but rarely used: the Scampering Dog, the Gaelic Edispunwod, and the Blumenbach positions.

12. When this position is used and the man supports himself by leaning his shoulders and back against a wall and the woman moves herself by pushing her feet against the wall, it is called "suspended congress" by Vatsyayana in *Kama Sutra*. Suspended congress uses more energy than most reclining positions, but not as much as Clasping the Tree and walking or doing knee bends.

13. You may get some ideas from the following books: Hector Boece and George Buchanan, *The Big Book of Sexual Positions*, (Newgate: Rank Publishers, 1982); Alex Comfort, *The New Joy of Sex* (NY: Crown Publishers, 1991); Thomas J. Wise, *The Illustrated Victorian Sex Manual*, (Marshalsea: Stews and Bagnios, 1889); and Merda Jakes, *1001 Ways to Do It* (Drury Lane Imprints, 1978).

14. Very.

15. Thus, some religions prohibit dancing because it leads one astray. On the other hand, some religions incorporate dancing as an integral part of worship for a similar reason; repeated rhythmic movement can induce a trance-like state (in which one may be closer to God, Terpsichore, Oneness or whatever).

16. See Chapter 6 for suggestions about choosing the appropriate music for Swell-Wimp.

17. My friends the Baileys recommended to me a Web site, Gala Balls. Assuming the site focused on society balls, I logged on to www.galaballs.com while writing this section on dancing. Imagine my surprise. It's a porn site. And they require a registration fee before you can enter.

18. For a fascinating discussion of the role of tubs in ancient and modern intercourse, see Dean Swift's *A Tale of a Tub* (London: John Nutt, 1973).

19. "Studies show that the combined use of both your upper and lower body during exercise burns more calories in less time. Unlike exercise bikes, treadmills and stair-climbers that only work your lower body…" (*The New Yorker*, April 16, 1991, Nordic Row TBX advertisement).

20. This is the "return-to-the-womb" phenomenon written about by Sigmund Freud, Carl Jung, Buster Crabb, and Wilhelm Reich.

21. The fat mass of the female breasts contributes additional flotational effect.

22. Here we are referring to common push-ups (one person). In order to do sexual push-ups even in shallow water, the lower partner will have to use a snorkel.

23. Snorkels solve this problem, although you will be under water only a brief time and you can hold your breath.

24. Incidentally, if you are bed-ridden (temporarily or permanently), you can use the hoisting bar to do pull-ups during intercourse or oral sex. Also, the cables, weights and pulleys used for placing limbs in traction can be used to increase the number of calories you expend during SexEx. Tie the cables to your waist, legs, shoulders and other body parts to make movement of those parts more difficult.

25. Or you can rent it inexpensively. Purchasing scuba gear just for underwater SexEx is not recommended unless (1) you and your partner are very determined, (2) you have ready access to deep water, and (3) you are financially well-off.

26. Goose bumps are also known as goose pimples and goose flesh.

27. During a discussion of goosebumps in Thomas Mann's *The Magic Mountain*, Hans Castorp notes that other things besides cold, such as hearing beautiful music or "a slate-pencil run across a pane of glass," can cause goosebumps. Dr. Behrens answers that the "body doesn't give a hang for the content of the stimulus. It may be minnows, it may be the Holy Ghost, the sebaceous glands are erected just the same".[b] Thus, instead of lowering the temperature of the room in order to induce goosebumps, you could play a recording of fingernails being scraped across a blackboard or a hyena's call or something similar. We don't recommend this because any sound annoying or frightening enough to raise goosebumps would probably also kill sexual desire.

28. Sensory perception can be so diminished that it can be dangerous. The Lackawanna County Coroner concluded that the deaths of a couple at the Taylor (Pennsylvania) Railroad Yards was due to diminished sensory awareness and lack of common sense (*The Scranton Tribune*, 31 June 1987, 5).

29. Low-calorie of course. Simple ice water is best, but not too much or your SexEx will be interrupted by cramps or trips to the bathroom.

30. See Introduction, note 8.

31. Most people believe deer to be harmless animals but they can be mean, even dangerous. They are like Gary Larson's cows. When people are watching they act like characters from *Bambi*, but at other times they will go out of their way to destroy vegetable and flower gardens. Bucks will come out of the forest, cross open fields, and avoid watch dogs in order to rub their antlers on newly planted young trees, destroying the bark and causing them to die. Deer will lie in wait alongside roads, hid in bushes, and perch on embankments in order to attack passing cars. And what about all the missing children, the faces on milk cartons? Scientists claimed that thalidomide was harmless, that organisms couldn't live in rocks hundreds of feet below the earth's surface and that stomach ulcers were caused by stress. And scientists insist that deer aren't sufficiently intelligent to plan and carry out the abductions of children. Think about it.

32. For more on the benefits and problems of fresh-air SexAct, see Adelaida and Ivan Veen, *Ardor in Ardis* (np: Cunnus-Coglione Books, 1923).

33. See Chapter 3, note 6.

34. Of course, the "active" partner can engage in vocalization also, although after forty or fifty sit-ups or leg lifts, he or she may be a bit "winded."

35. We have recently had a "feeler" from a group of investors who would like to open a chain of Swell-Wimp Hotel-Gyms. Designed in strict accordance with the results of our study, these would provide hotel-like accommodations (cold and hot rooms, a selection of beds, etc.), gymnasium-like facilities (specially designed equipment and clothing), medical services, and trained aides to help you get the most of your Swell-Wimp experience. By the time you read this, one may be located in your area. I can't tell you what to look for in the yellow pages, because we haven't chosen a name yet. Since Dr. Flanders is no longer associated with the Swell-Wimp Project (as it is now called), there could be no objection to using my name.

36. *Thus Spake Zarathustra: A Book for All and None*, trans. Walter Kaufmann (Harmondsworth: Penguin Books, 1954), 78.

Chapter 11

1. Q. Waite and I. Racque, *A Case Study: Warba & Bubiyan After the Attacks* (Berlin: Waswill Dasweib, 1992).

2. Given the fact that intellectually and maturationally, most men remain at the 14-year-old level, it is probably a good thing that they do not return to the plateau level as do women, since the frustration resulting from being aroused but physiologically unable to satisfy their arousal might have led to the suicidal extinction of the species long ago. Women over the centuries have become accustomed to being aroused but unsatisfied. C. F.

3. *The Hite Report* (NY: Macmillan; London: Collier Macmillan, 1976), 86.

4. We are aware that arguing by analogy is always suspect; however, see George Tylutki, "An Invalid But Useful Analogy," *Computer Language*, July 1991, 119–120.

5. Therefore, you should be careful about lunch-time SexEx if you do strenuous physical labor.

6. You can talk about anything. You might want to engage in post-coital assessment at this time or defer it to later (see Chapter 6). You can talk "love talk," tell jokes, or even discuss your plans for the next day. This is a good time to get to know your partner better.

7. Actually, tissues are not as good as towels because they come apart easily; it is not pleasant to pick dried tissue flecks from a flaccid penis.

8. Vatsyayana advises eating some betel leaves to sweeten the mouth after intercourse.

Chapter 12

1. Vatsyayana considered this aspect of SexAct so important that he included the culinary arts (not just cooking) as one of the major subjects to be studied by cultured, desirable women.

2. Non-alcoholic. Alcoholic beverages cloud the senses, decrease sexual desire, and are high in calories.

3. Remember, low-calorie; for example, dried prunes (no syrup) or doofekaf, the delicious low-calorie Bulgarian pastry.

4. As the Romans used to say, "*fabas indulcet fames*"; that is, even beans taste good when you're hungry.

5. *Everything You Always Wanted to Know About Sex But Were Afraid to Ask* (NY: Bantam Books, 1969).

6. Thus, it is very popular with men, whose egos are "fragile." C. F.

7. From chilies are made an analgesic cream for cluster headaches, a treatment for shingles and a salve for phantom-limb pain.

8. Poppies, Satyrion, Argumentum Tripodium and Apicius are also ineffective.

9. We are aware of a couple for whom borsch is an aphrodisiac, not because it has any inherent power to increase sexual desire, but because they had borsch for dinner the evening they first engaged in (very satisfactory) coitus. Thus, they engage in gustatory foreplay. For an excellent discussion of the power of the mind (to heal) see Walter A. Brown, "The Placebo Effect," *Scientific American* (January 1998, 90–95).

10. John Barth coined this term in his book about nautical sex, *Tidewater Tales* (NY: G. P. Putnam's Sons, 1987). When a woman's vagina becomes moist with secretions due to sexual stimulation, she is lushing.

11. I recently heard a report on WEZX-FM (Scranton, PA) about a beverage, "Prunetang," specifically designed for SexEx as Gatorade is designed for sports activity, but I have not had time to verify its efficacy. Reportedly, it smells like tuna fish and tastes like cranberries. P. B.

12. This fact has been known for centuries. In Shakespeare's *Macbeth* (Act 2, scene 3) Macduff asks "What three things does drink especially provoke?" The porter answers, "Marry, sir, nose-painting, sleep and urine. Lechery, sir, it provokes and unprovokes: it provokes the desire, but it takes away the performance. Therefore, much drink may be said to be an equivocator with lechery: it makes him, and it mars him; it sets him on, and it takes him off; it persuades him, and disheartens him; makes him stand to, and not stand to: in conclusion, equivocates him in a sleep, and giving him the lie, leaves him."

13. Since smoking is such a deleterious habit and one very difficult to break, you might ask why we have not studied the possibility of using SexAct to stop smoking. We haven't because (it is clear to us) the very powerful tobacco lobby is working behind the scenes to prevent us from obtaining funding.

14. Even though, as we pointed out earlier, our senses of smell and taste are diminished when we are sexually aroused.

15. Money is odorless. [ed.]

16. Although, if the vagina becomes too wet, it can be coated with honey to increase friction. It is harmless, washes off easily, and smells and tastes good.

17. Generally, women have a better sense of smell, but men respond to smells as attractors better. Thus, perfumes are generally worn by women.

18. Of course, the opposite may also be true. Some people are unable to eat capons and crabs, not because they do not like the taste, but because of unpleasant associations. If you have this problem, you might want to consult *Overcoming Food Aversions* by Andrei Chikatilo (Moscow: Lutumilious Books, 1991).

19. I find the smell of vanilla extract very nice and the smell of celery makes me hungry. Thus, I avoid celery and celery powder during SexEx, but I like my partner to daub a little vanilla on her body. P. B.

20. What is poison to some, is food to others. [ned]

21. The word phallic is Greek in origin and refers to anything that resembles an erect phallus (the penis). Yonic is Sanskrit in origin and refers to anything that resembles the vulva (external female genitalia). For Hindus, the phallus (or lingam) is the symbol of the god Shiva and the yoni is the symbol of the goddess Shakti; thus, their religious symbolism has at its center the union of the male and female.

Chapter 13

1. *The New Joy of Sex* (NY: Crown Publishers, 1991). We have been unable to find anything about Erlen.

2. Incidentally, Swell-Wimp is unrelated to GUIs (Graphical User Interfaces for computers) which are composed of WIMPs (Windows, Icons, Menus, and Pointing devices).

3. Reportedly, Condomania in Greenwich Village, New York sells over 200 kinds of condoms. Most drug stores don't carry such a variety, but you should be able to find one you like.

4. It is especially important to be wary if your relationship has lasted several to many years. Statistically, there is a much greater chance of one partner "cheating" in a seven-year marriage than there is in a one-year affair, because of boredom, dissatisfaction, and animosities that have built up over a long time. (There is truth in the old notion of the "seven-year itch.") In a one-year old relationship the partners are frequently still "in love" and idealistic. The most dangerous time for "cheating" is between the fifth and twenty-second years.

5. I will admit that I may be a bit biased, since as a college professor I have lots of time between classes and committee meetings for interesting exercise, Swell-Wimp and other energy-expending activities.

6. Our study participants favored the Fealy Econopedic mattress; it is firm and inexpensive.

7. Emily Dickinson preferred a big bed in a dark room (Poem 829):

> Ample make this Bed—
> Make this Bed with Awe—
> In it wait till Judgment break
> Excellent and Fair.
> Be its Mattress straight—
> Be its Pillow round—
> Let no Sunrise' yellow noise
> Interrupt this Ground—

8. Beds have been so important throughout history that they often appear as specific items in wills. For example, Shakespeare left his second-best bed to his wife in his will. See E. A. J. Honigmann, "The Second-best Bed," *The New York Review of Books*, 7 November 1991, 27–30.

9. Incidentally, my niece says that when you "make the bed" you should be sure to put the open sides of the pillow cases toward the edges of the bed (not toward the center). Then, when the pillow monsters come out at night, they will fall on the floor. Isn't that precious? Of course, the sounds of the monsters hitting the floor may disturb your sleep. Alternatively, you can place both open ends toward each other and then when the pillow monsters run out of one pillow they run directly into the other. They're not very bright, but eventually they may figure out what you've done, and then your sleep may be disrupted by their grumblings. P. B.

10 It is a scandal that so many people in this country do not even have a bedroom, let alone two bedrooms. Before you go to the trouble and expense of furnishing a second bedroom, you might want to think about donating the time and money to a charity. You will help others and increase your own self-esteem. C. F.

11. Of course, a cheaper alternative is to raise the bed by placing something under its legs. Just be sure that the bed is secure and stable; you do not want it to suddenly jolt downward or even collapse under you.

12. In the lab we found it convenient to simply attach a paper towel holder to the bed's headboard. You might want to try this.

13. Dr. Helen Caldicott points out that we don't inherit the earth from our ancestors, but borrow it from our descendants. C. F.

14. The driver of the vehicle should never engage in SexAct while the vehicle is moving! Even mutual masturbation, although popular, is dangerous. And no form of SexAct should be attempted on a moving motorcycle.

15. There was a joke in the 1950s: how you can identify a car owned by a teenager? It doesn't have arm rests on the doors in the back because they hurt your head.

16. Incidentally, all of this is true for SexAct in a rocking chair also. It sounds nice, but you have to be quite limber to find any pleasure in it.

17. Frank S. Caprio in *The Sexually Adequate Female* (NY: The Citadel Press, 1953) claims that some women are so "frigid" as to be able to read a book while their "husbands take their pleasure" (67). See Chapter 14 for our view of Caprio's views. C. F.

18. This is true despite that fact that our sense of hearing diminishes during sexual arousal. Like Pavlov's dogs, we have become so conditioned to acting when the telephone rings that we react even when we can barely hear it and have much better things to do.

19. Phone etiquette seems to have disappeared. How often have you answered the phone and heard a voice say, "Who's this?" It's usually a wrong number and the caller doesn't recognize your voice. I am repeatedly astounded (and angered) by the arrogance and ignorance of such people. Can you imagine opening your door and having the person who rang your doorbell ask "Who're you?"! Is it so difficult to understand that when you place a call and the person answers "Hello," you should identify yourself. For example, when I call my co-author to discuss this book and I don't recognize the voice of the person who answers the phone I say something like: "This is Dr. Thomas. May I speak to Dr. Jacobs please?" And these wrong-number people get so angry when I try to teach them the correct way to use a phone! See also Mark Caldwell, *A Short History of Rudeness* (NY: Picador, 1999).

20. In many ways a hotel or motel room is an excellent location for Swell-Wimp. The mattresses usually aren't very good, but a bathroom with clean towels is nearby. You can turn up the heating or cooling depending upon your preference. Someone else will clean up after you. You can get away from the kids and other distractions and achieve privacy for a few hours. Some hotels and motels rent by the hour and X-rated visual stimulation is available for those who like/need it. Some hotels and motels will even provide a partner (at additional cost, of course).

21. New York: Random House, 1992. Before the invention of the telephone, people sometimes engaged in epistolary sex. For example William Thackeray tells us that Sir Pitt Crawley "screwed his tenants by letter" (*Vanity Fair*, 1848; Penguin Books, 1968, 471).

22. Of course, if you really want a mobile "pleasure palace," you can purchase a small Winnebago-type vehicle. Or you can convert a used ambulance (the large truck-chassis type) or a step-van (bread/potato chip truck) whose aluminum bodies never

rust. We don't recommend the type of camper that fits into a pickup truck (not enough room, you can't get from the camper to the cab without going outside, and they're ugly) or camper trailers (they take too long to set up).

23. Vatsyayana calls this the "pleasure room" and recommends decorating it with flowers, perfumes and a "pot for spitting." We agree.

24. Rachel P. Maines' *The Technology of Orgasm* (The Johns Hopkins Univ. Press, 1999) is a fascinating account of the history of the vibrator. It was designed to save physicians the labor of digitally bringing their female to climax. They treated female hysteria (basically women who were sexually unsatisfied and sufficiently wealthy to do something about it; taking on a lover was no guarantee of sexual satisfaction) by inducing hysterical paroxysm, a euphemism for orgasm. Incidentally, a saber saw (without blade) and orbital sander (without sandpaper) are inexpensive and readily available substitutes for vibrators; use the appropriately-shaped part of the tool's plastic body.

25. In Poem 358 Dickinson says that she found nothing to fear in intercourse, except the UTIs to which she was susceptible: "[I] Dread, but the Whizzing."

Chapter 14

1. By "older people" we mean those who are older because of chronological age. We can find no better term. The *Quarterly Review of Doublespeak* (April 1993, 5) reported that the American Association of Retired Persons intended to use the term "geriatrics" instead of "chronologically gifted." We find both terms silly as we do "seniors" and "senior citizens."

2. *Sexual Behavior in the Human Male* (Philadelphia and London: W. B. Saunders, 1948), 204.

3. *The Decameron*, trans. Richard Aldington (NY: Dell Publishing, 1930), 249. None of the participants in our study was older than 32.

4. I must admit that I was blind to the truth of Boccaccio's statement. I assumed, as so many people do, that grandparents weren't interested in sex. When Dr. Flanders became a grandmother at age 38, I realized that my views of old age and grandparentage were out of synch with reality. So I decided to add this chapter which is based on research of the literature and interviews with seven older people (aged 59 to 91). Because the population of the United States is growing older and because health care costs are exploding and because almost one billion dollars is spend annually for

funding research on aging, we believe that we may be able to obtain funding for a study of Swell-Wimp and older people. P. B.

5. Harvey L. and Jean S. Gochros, *The Sexually Oppressed* (NY: Associated Press, 1977), 1.

6. The statistics are a bit misleading because the improvement has generally resulted from reducing the number of childhood deaths, not from people living longer than their ancestors. Still, this means that many more people are living to old age. C. F.

7. Of course, people of any age may be physically limited. It was only after we had received the galleys of this book that it was pointed out to us that we do not address the subject of Swell-Wimp and the handicapped. The only thing that we can say at this point is that most of Swell-Wimp can be adapted for use by those with physical limitations. This is another subject that we will add to our list of topics to be investigated when we obtain funding.

8. You may also want to read some of the following: Dee Ann Green Birkel and Susan Birkel Freitag, *Forever Fit: A Step-By-Step Guide for Older Adults* (NY: Plenum Publishing, 1991); *Sexual Anarchy: Gender and Culture at the Fin de Siècle* by Elaine Showalter (NY: Penguin USA, 1991); Harvey L. and Jean S. Gochros, *The Sexually Oppressed* (New York: Associated Press, 1977); *One Hundred Years After Tomorrow* ed. and trans. Darlene J. Sadlier (Indiana UP, 1991); K. Heslinga *Not Made of Stone: The Sexual Problems of Handicapped People* (Springfield, Illinois: Charles C. Thomas, 1974).

9. Bertram Copeland Rumfoord's *Sex and Athletics for the Senior Male* (Ilium, NY: Dresden Books, 1945) does not incorporate the latest nutritional information but contains excellent advice for men over sixty-five.

10. *Not Made of Stone* (Springfield, Illinois: Charles C. Thomas, 1974), 93.

11. We are not familiar with the Sexercise Tolerance Test but it sounds appropriate. In fact, wearing the monitors will increase your energy output during SexAct.

12. See Chapter 9 for more on birth control.

13. Alex Comfort in *Joy of Sex* (NY: Crown Publishers, 1991) reports that rectal intercourse was a common practice in the nineteenth century among the working class as a method of birth control.[a]

14. David Reuben in *Everything You always Wanted to Know About Sex But Were Afraid to Ask* (NY: Bantam Books, 1969) points out that childhood and old age are the times when sexual feelings are present but the means to satisfy them are not; therefore, these are the times when people engage in masturbation most

often. Masturbation is a frequent method of sexual release for older and handicapped people.

15. *Sexual Behavior in the Human Female* (Philadelphia and London: W. B. Saunders, 1953), 262–263.

16. Most modern jails are being designed much differently from in the past. The trend is away from rows of cells with steel bars for doors and on the windows and toward mingling the prisoners and guards. This trend is, in part, stimulated by cost; it is cheaper to build prisons without lots of steel and locks. The interesting thing is that the incidence of violence and vandalism is greatly reduced (*Morning Edition*, National Public Radio, 14 April 1993).

17. Ronald Reagan didn't let his age or attitudes prevent him from becoming President and it certainly isn't the reason his was such a bad administration. He was a lazy, mental light-weight his entire life. His age simply made it more acceptable (or expected) for him to be sleepy and dopey.[b]

18. Sure, you slow down a little but you shouldn't act like a dotty old fool. Today no one expects you to sit in a rocking chair on the porch. There is no excuse for standing around slack-mouthed (you can't all be ill with the few physical and mental illnesses that can cause this).

19. As of 1977, 95% of people over 65 lived in the community (not in an institution), 81% got around by themselves and 30% were still working (*The Sexually Oppressed*, 5).

20. *The Sexually Oppressed,* 29–30. But if you have a condition that could result in sudden death, you should advise your partner. Stephen King in *Gerald's Game* (NY: Viking, 1992) chronicles what can happen when you do not properly consider the effect of your sudden death upon your partner.

21. You don't have to be old to have arthritis. Swell-Wimp is good for arthritics of any age who are of age.

22. "The Healing Powers of Sex" by Kristin von Kreisler in *Reader's Digest*, June 1993, 17; reprinted from *Redbook*, April 1993.

23. William H. Masters, Virginia E. Johnson and Robert C. Kolodny, *On Sex and Human Loving* (Boston & Toronto: Little, Brown and Co., 1982), 185.

24. Of course, common sense rules. Satisfying an urge by having SexAct with someone who has a venereal disease can result in problems greater than not satisfying the sexual desire. The long-term problems that result from a 14-year-old male satisfying his sexual desires by impregnating a 14-year-old girl generally outweigh the short-term benefits.

25. Von Kreisler, 19. I find that orgasm will eliminate headache pain for about 45 minutes, during which time I am able to fall asleep. C. F.

26. By limited financial resources, we mean "poor." We do not mean a "fixed income," which is often cited as a problem for older people. Social Security and many retirement payments are indexed to inflation. If inflation goes up, there is an increase in the benefits. This is NOT a fixed income. Most people who work for minimum wage have fixed incomes. No matter how hard they work or how high inflation goes, they will not see an increase in their pays. People who work under a contract (like teachers) have a fixed income for the life of the contract. They will not get larger pay checks because inflation increases or their kids need shoes. And they have no special expectations that they will receive more under the next contract (and justified fears that they will receive less). Most active workers must get a different or second job to increase their incomes. Most retired people can count on a (small) yearly increase in benefits.

27. I have an older friend who has almost totally lost her ability to remember short-term. You might imagine that she would find it very frustrating, but she seems quite happy, meeting and making friends with the same people each day. C. F.

28. I have never had a good memory, especially for names, and now that I've passed the half-century mark, my memory is even less reliable.[c] I have a busy life and find it tremendously annoying when my short-term memory fails me—when I have to waste time looking for my car keys, for example. So I have covered a baseball cap with Velcro and attached Velcro strips to my key ring, pipe and tobacco pouch, pen, TV remote control, pen and other objects. When I'm through using them, I slap them on my hat. Now I only have to remember where I left my hat. You may want to try something similar such as putting Velcro strips on the front of your shirt or blouse. This won't directly help you find a sexual partner, but it will reduce the number of things you have to worry about. P. B.

29. Alfred C. Kinsey, Wardell B. Pomeroy and Clyde E. Martin, *Sexual Behavior in the Human Male* (Philadelphia & London: W. B. Saunders, 1948), 235.

30. As Virgil says in the *Aeneid* about aged Priam's "spear", "*telum imbelle sine ictu*" (A feeble weapon without a thrust).

31. Milton Berle, who is over eighty years old, says, "I enjoy sex, especially the one in winter."

32. Interestingly, **fear** of impotence can occur at any age, but may, in fact, be more common in men of 45–50 than in men of 65–75 who have adjusted to the changes that come with age.

33. Our favorite poet writes about her second sexual experience with a semi-impotent lawyer (Poem 190):

> He was weak, and I was strong—then—
> So He let me lead him in—
> ....
> He strove—and I strove—too—
> We didn't do it—tho'!

34. Even someone as sensitive as Dickinson was misinformed about the relative commonness of impotence (Poem 287):

> Geneva's farthest skill
> Can't put the puppet bowing—
> That just now dangled still—
> ....
> It will not stir for Doctors—
> This Pendulum of snow—

Notice her disparagement of the penis as a "puppet" and a cold "pendulum."

35. There is some dispute about the origin of the word "impotent." Most dictionaries claim *lucus a non lucendo* that it is a combination of the prefix "im" (Latin for 'not') and "potens" (Scottish from Latin for 'have power'). However, Ian McMack in **Gaelic Etymologies** (New York: J. S. G. Boggs, 1990) claims it is a combination of "imp" (from Middle English from Old English from Common Romance from Latin for 'small demon') and "o" (Scottish for 'of') and "gent" (Middle English from Old French from Latin for 'to beget'); thus, "imp o'gent" for "demon of the [my] begetter."

36. This was a problem with Emily Dickinson's first lover, a teamster who felt guilty about cheating on his wife (Poem 359):

> I gained it so—
> ....
> It hung so high
> As well the Sky
> ....
> I said I gained it—
> This—was all—
> Look, how I clutch it

Lest it.1 fall—

37. As Leonid Nemoicheck wrote in his recent book, *In Search of the Perfect Orgasm*, "It's better to copulate than never" (Hafen: Momzer & Sons, 1989), 96.

38. Diabetes is one of the few illnesses that can directly cause impotence; it's 2–5 times more common in male diabetics than in the general population. Further, it can be permanent (Gochros, 31).

39. Studies done by Mary F. Dallman of the University of California at San Francisco have shown that stress can cause "the redistribution of energy stores from muscle to fat, particularly abdominal fat, [which] may have a role in the development of abdominal obesity, which is strongly associated with increased incidence of adult-onset diabetes, coronary artery disease and stroke" (Kristin Leutwyler, "Don't Stress", *Scientific American*, January 1998, 30). As we indicated earlier, obesity itself can cause impotence. So, stress can cause obesity, obesity can cause impotence and impotence can cause stress. Another vicious circle.

40. Masters, Johnson and Kolodny report that (1) there has been no surge of impotence corresponding to the spread of feminism; (2) male partners of women with full-time careers outside the home actually have lower rates of impotence than the male partners of traditional housewives; and (3) more "masculine" women are as sexually responsive and satisfied as more "feminine" women (*On Sex and Human Loving*, 451). C. F.

41. In a study of 1300 males, 40 to 70 years old, nearly 90% who ranked high on a measurement for depression reported moderate or complete impotence (T. Adler, "Impotence: More Than a Middle-age Metaphor," **Science News**, 8 January 1994, 21). In this same study it was discovered that heart patients who smoked were almost three times more likely to suffer total impotence than those who did not.

42. Gochros claims that there is really no such thing as a male menopause; the decrease in the male hormone testosterone occurs very gradually as men grow older. Reubens, however, uses the term and notes that it is more gradual and, therefore, harder to detect than female menopause.

43. Although this is changing as more women take up smoking more and larger numbers of women enter stressful occupations. Also, see "Problems: Females" later in the chapter.

44. Physiological impotence is usually due to tiredness and less often to a deficiency of testosterone. Injections can help, but the pituitary gland regulates the distribution of testosterone, so sometimes when men are given injections, the pituitary "thinks" everything is OK and tells the adrenals and testicles to stop working, and

they atrophy. The testicles, adrenals and pituitary glands cannot be exercised except by engaging in SexAct.

45. That "magical gewgaw" as Nabokov calls it in *Ada* (NY: McGraw-Hill, 1960), 420.

46. An excellent narrative about the heartbreak of impotence can be found in Peter Resurgam's book *Damaged Goods* (Paris: Eugène Brieux, 1903).

47. Words of wisdom from the cover of that helpful compendium of galactic knowledge (including sexual), *The Hitchhiker's Guide to the Galaxy* by Douglas Adams (NY: Pocket Books, 1979).

48. Thanks to Viagra, many men who thought their sex lives had come to an end can now become Swell-Wimpers. Tell your older, male friends about this book. P. B.

Once again scientists, who claim to know what they're doing (genetically-engineered food, for example), have stumbled upon a "breakthrough." Viagra's ability to creating a usable erection is a side-effect of a drug designed for another purpose. The researchers had no idea it would happen, just as they did not know that a heart medication would cause ear hair to grow; that side effect became Rogaine. {Jerry, 2 notes above: "the heartbreak of impotence." You've got to be kidding!} C. F.

49. *Consumer Reports*, May 1993, 300.

50. Von Kreisler, 17–18.

51. So 40% of all women **do** experience "remarkable physical or emotional symptoms." It seems likely that much more funding would be made available for research on menopause if 40% of all men experienced similar "change-of-life" symptoms (see the next note). C. F.

52. Some of the other effects of decreased estrogen are: hot flashes, shifting of fat deposits, increased wrinkling of the skin, dryness of the hair, atrophy of the breasts, increased facial hair, deepening voice, coarsened features, gradual baldness, depression, irritability, insomnia and decreased protection against heart disease.

53. Frigidity is a pejorative term and should be replaced by "orgasmic impairment." As with men there is a range of impairment and it is usually psychological in origin. C. F.

54. Dickinson wrote in Poem 880 about a telegraph operator's ability to bring her to climax only occasionally:

> The rose content may bloom
> But if the Lady come[s]
> But once a Century, the Rose
> Superfluous become[s]—

55. Those who write about "sex" too often assume that their readers are well-educated and well-informed. This topic of frigidity may seem old (Caprio's book was published in 1953); it may seem that it doesn't need to be covered, but there are pockets of ignorance (sometimes as large as an entire state) in the U.S. If one is going to assume everyone knows that the post-World War 2 notion of frigidity is gender-driven nonsense, then one might as well assume: that "everyone knows" that trickle-down economics is, in fact, voodoo economics; that blacks are not genetically inferior; that sending rockets into space does not cause it to rain at your house; that sitting on a cold rock will not give you hemorrhoids; that when your nose itches someone is not necessarily talking about you; that a defendant is found "not guilty" not "innocent"; that the cover-up is worse than the crime; that Freudian psychology is just so much bosh[d]; and that just because it's in print doesn't mean that it's true (else "they" couldn't print it). Does everyone know these things?

56. Gochros says the clitoris may be slightly reduced in size as women age (probably due to a general reduction in body fat and size), but Reuben says there may be enlargement of the clitoris (probably due to hormonal changes).

57. The term "hysterectomy" is derived from the Greek *hustera* meaning "womb." This is the same root of "hysteria"; it was thought that only women could be "hysterical"—a condition caused by disturbances of the uterus. C. F.

58. *Sexual Behavior in the Human Female* (Philadelphia & London: W. B. Saunders, 1953), 353.

59. On Sex and Human Loving, 170.

60. While many women fear a "change-of-life" baby, others experience an increase in sexual drive after menopause because the fear of pregnancy disappears.

61. We feel that there is entirely too much emphasis placed upon breasts in our culture. However, we cannot change society. The decision about whether to undergo reconstructive surgery must be made by each woman, in conjunction with her physician and her partner(s).

62. See Chapters 5 and 8.

63. Every woman has a supplier of testosterone in the adrenal glands which is why reduced estrogen production causes masculinization.

64. See also *Living with the Glacier* by Kholod Golod (National Geographical Society, 1990).

65. Von Kreisler, 19.

66. However, see Reverend Billy C. Wirtz, *The Missionary Position* (Raleigh, NC: np, 1993) for a spirited defense of the face-to-face, lying-down position, especially

for obese people. Christopher Hitchens' *The Missionary Position* (London & NY: Verso, 1996) is about Mother Teresa, not sexual positions.

67. King Edward VII, who was very fat, had a special couch resembling a gynecological table made to enable him to engage in intercourse. Clearly he was a man in need of Swell-Wimp if ever there was one. C. F.

68. See "Clasping the Tree" in Chapter 10 for more positions.

69. For more on visually stimulating foods, see *The Lickerish Licorice* by Lewis Cibber and Colley Theobald [no relation] (Calliope, NJ: Paronomasia Ltd., 1969).

70. "Can We Live To 150?" *Popular Science*, November 1993, 77–82.

71. "Can We Live To 150?" 77–81.

72. Quitting smoking is the best thing you can do to extend your life.

73. There is a slightly alcoholic beverage which Eastern Europeans claim helps sustain an active sex life: Elder Berrywine. I don't know what this is made from or how it is made, but there is sufficient anecdotal evidence of its effectiveness that research funds should be made available to investigation it.

74. "Can You Live Longer?" *Consumer Reports*, January 1992, 7–15.

75. "Can We Live to 150?" 82.

76. *Time of Our Lives: The Science of Human Aging* (NY: Oxford Univ. Press, 1999).

77. *A Means to an End: The Biological Basis of Aging and Death* (NY: Oxford Univ. Press, 1999).

78. "Can You Live Longer?" Notice that "scientists" have given us conflicting advice. On the one hand, severely restricting caloric intake which will result in a minimum body weight *might* extend your life. On the other hand, it is natural and *probably* desirable to gain weight as you age. In the January 1998 issue of *Consumer Reports* in a review of diet books, we find that Robert Atkins advises eliminating nearly all carbohydrates from your diet because they ultimately raise the blood-insulin level, a bad thing. However, Robert Arnot advises eating foods that require a lot of chewing and resist digestion, such as high-fiber cereals, because as they are absorbed they raise the blood-insulin level, which is desirable. As we've pointed out before, you must be vigilantly skeptical whenever you read about dieting, exercise, weight loss and weight maintenance.

79. When you go grocery shopping do not behave in a stereotypical manner. Keep your cart on the right side of the aisle (in the United States). Don't lean on your cart as if it were a walker with wheels; stand up straight and push your cart in front of you. If you have a disability and have difficulty walking, stay on the right side of the aisle out of the way; do not travel down the center at a snail's pace. As you move from aisle to aisle, do not round off the corners; this invariably causes you to run into someone

or causes a traffic jam. Do not just walk away from your cart to search for some product, unless you have properly parked your cart. In short, do not assume that age brings with it the privilege to act like a nincompoop.

This brings to mind something else that annoys me. Every supermarket seems to arrange its products in a different, and as far as I can tell, random order. Why aren't the products shelved in alphabetical order?

80. See Madeleine Proust, "Diet and the Elderly Neurasthenic," *The Chirurgical Journal*, 56: 237–252.

81. In New York City, you can be fellated for as little as $2–$5. This not the type of sexual activity we advocate, because being fellated by a streetwalker will not help you to lose weight and consorting with streetwalkers increases your risk of contracting and transmitting a disease.

82. Garcia Gabriel Marquez writes about living alone for a long time in *100 Years of Solitude* (trans. Gregory Rabassa [NY: Avon Books, 1970]) as does Elena Bonner in *Alone Together* (NY: A. A. Knopf, 1986).

83. Reuben claims that if sexual activity is interrupted for sixty days or more, statistically, sexual activity will not resume. Both men and women can masturbate to keep things going when their partners are temporarily unavailable.

84. If you cannot get out, you may need to contact an organization that specializes in providing sexual partners for the home bound.

85. In 1990 Americans spent an estimated $3 to $4-billion for cosmetic surgery and another billion dollars on moisturizers ("Can You Live Longer?").

86. And often it is blue! It seems unlikely that anyone except Superman could be attracted to a woman with blue hair.

87. This may not seem important, but you should ask yourself why coitus is frequently referred to as "a piece of ass."

88. W. B. Yeats, "Sailing to Byzantium," line 10 and William Wordsworth, *The Prelude*, line 459.

89. If your partner is turned off by the sight of your body, you don't have to get naked for Swell-Wimp.

90. Nancy Reagan, who clearly is old and not attractive, maintained her appearance and kept her sexual partner through careful attention to diet and dress. She provides a fascinating look at elder-presidential-sex in an interview in the Japanese magazine *Shufo no Tomo* (The Housewife's Friend), January 1982.

91. Vladimir Nabokov, in his moving chronicle of the case of Humbert Humbert, shows that a large difference in age between partners doesn't reduce sexual pleasure, but that there are social pressures which may.

92. For example, in the following 15 famous May-December relationships only three women are older than the men: Mohammed was 15 years older than his wife; Sam Donaldson is 22 years older than his wife; Dolly was 17 years younger than President Madison; Dick Smothers is 20 years older than his wife Lorraine; Michael was 20 years older than Isabel; T. S. Eliot was 38 years older than Valerie Fletcher; 40 years separated Alfred Stieglitz and his wife Dorothy Norman; Alan Thicke is 22 years older than his wife Gina Tolleson; Mike Todd was older than Elizabeth Taylor by 23 years; Anna Nicole Smith was 26 years younger than J. Howard Marshall; there is a 34-year difference between Rod and Paula Steiger; Annette Bening is 37 years younger than Warren Beatty; Ed McMahon is 40 years older than his wife Paula; Rosanne was 14 years older than her husband Ben Thomas; Elizabeth Taylor is (was?) 20 years older than Larry Fortensky; and Janie Woods was 12 years older than her husband Tea Cake.

93. As it has been since at least 411 BC when Aristophanes' *Lysistrata* was first performed: "When a man comes home [from war], no matter how grey he is, he soon finds a girl to marry. But a woman's bloom is short and fleeting; if she doesn't grasp her chance, no man is willing to marry her…" (from *The Norton Anthology of World Masterpieces*, Maynard Mack and others, eds., 2 vols., 4th ed. [New York: W. W. Norton, 1979] 2: 501.)

94. Anne, I'm unable to locate the source (Von Kreisler?) of this quotation. Do you have it in your notes?

Chapter 15

1. See Appendix A.

2. Women's Network: www.ivillage.com

3. Kristin von Kreisler, "The Healing Powers of Sex," *Reader's Digest*, June 1993, 18; reprinted from *Redbook*, April 1993.

4. *New York Magazine*, December 8, 1972 in *The Book of Lists*, David Wallenchinsky, Irving Wallace and Amy Wallace (NY: Bantam Books, 1977).

5. With a grain of salt. Limited funding and the publishing deadlines have prevented us from doing extensive follow-ups of each and every subject of our study. Now that the book is published, we hope to obtain additional information about long-term benefits.

6. Prologue to the Miller's Tale, *The Tales of Canterbury*, ed. Robert A. Pratt (Boston: Houghton Mifflin, 1974), l. 3186.

7. *The Decameron*, trans. Richard Aldington (NY: Dell, 1930), 639.

Appendix A

1. Of course, funding for research that benefits tobacco growers was not stopped.

2. See Anne Fausto-Sterling, "Why Do We Know So Little About Human Sex?" *Discover*, June 1992, 29–31. Fausto-Sterling, a professor of medical science at Brown University, argues for the recognition of five sexes rather than the traditional three. In addition to males, females and "herms" or hermaphrodites, there are "merms" or male pseudohermaphrodites (who have testes and some aspects of the female genitalia but no ovaries) and "ferms" or female pseudohermaphrodites (who have ovaries and some external male genitalia but lack testes). For more on this see *Popular Science*, September 1993, 37.

3. We've just heard that someone is planning to introduce RU-486 into the US, but we can provide no further information.

4. In the sense discussed in Chapter 2. There are, of course, some individuals who feel that sexual activity is work (unpleasant activity) and those for whom it is a profession.

5. *Sexual Behavior in the Human Male*, (Philadelphia & London: W. B. Saunders, 1948), 157.

6. It was our aim to be able to publish the results of scientific research not some populist nonsense based on some half-baked idea. This required that we purchase a number of exquisitely precise measuring instruments. Our decision to "be scientific" and our need to obtain the appropriate equipment resulted in more than half of our funding being used to purchase equipment even before we had begun to gather data.

7. An erg is a (centimeter-gram-second) unit of energy equal to the work done by a force of one dyne acting over a distance of one centimeter. A dyne is a measure of the force required to impart an acceleration of one centimeter per second per second to a mass of one gram. A joule is a unit of energy equal to the work done when a current of one amp is passed through a resistance of one ohm for one second. It is also equal to the work done when the point of application of force of one newton is displaced one meter in the direction of the force.

8. Some other units of measurement you may not be familiar with: a centimeter is 1/100 of a meter or .3937 inch. A meter is equal to 39.37 inches. A gram is one-thousandth of a kilogram which is 2.2046 pounds. A heptad is a metrical unit consisting of seven feet. A kilometer is equal to .62137 mile and a dynamometer is an instrument used to measure force or power. 9743 wits make up an academy. A newton is the unit of force required to accelerate a mass of one kilogram one meter per second or 100,000 dynes. Four noggins make a pint. An amp (ampere) is a unit of electric current that under controlled circumstances produces a force between two wires of 2 X 10-7 newtons per meter. A ton is 2000 pounds. A tun is four kilderkins. A pound is equal to 16 ounces or 7000 grams. An ounce is equal to 437.5 grams. The answer is 42. An ohm is a unit of electrical resistance equal to that of a conductor in which a current of one ampere is produced by a potential of one volt across its terminals. A volt is a sudden movement in fencing made to avoid a thrust.

9. National Institute of Hemiplegia, *Publication 217*, 1979, 23.

10. Early on we abandoned joules as a unit of measure of sexual activity because it made us laugh.

11. Control Data Corporation, Internal Memorandum (H.K. to J.D.), 23 May 1986.

12. A gram or small calorie is the quantity of heat required to raise the temperature of one gram of water one degree Centigrade from initial temperature (usually 3.98C, 14.5C or 19.5C) at one atmosphere pressure. There are also mean, kilogram and thermochemical calories. The last is equal to 4.184 joules.

13. Primarily, a calorimeter and a more powerful computer to which we could directly attach measuring devices. Since the new computer was not compatible with the first, we lost some time re-entering data.

14. In a recent study of how caterpillars moved and of their energy efficiency, the insects were actually placed on tiny treadmills! Clearly, some things are more easily done in the laboratory.

15. In this instance the subjects were engaging in coitus in the "missionary position."

16. Which Mr. Norbert did not find unpleasurable.

17. Insufficient funding prevented us from (1) bringing on board someone qualified to perform this procedure or (2) taking the subject to an institution where it could be performed. It is unlikely that we could have found a willing subject anyway (Louisa was not part of the study at this time).

18. Tumescent means swollen or enlarged; in reference to the penis it refers to an erection, a hard-on, a boner. In the detumescent state it is called many things, including dong, wiener, my-friend-Bob and so on.

19. Flaccid is a term derived from French and Latin and means limp, flabby, hanging (Bob is tired).

20. Except for Mr. Barville, but he had already had his penis pierced with a gold ring and a pearl pin which would interfere with our measurements.

21. This is as you would expect from professionals.

22. Of course, you are familiar with the Heisenberg effect, but you may not know that William Wordsworth, in his poem "Tables Turned," anticipated Heisenberg by many years when he wrote, "we murder to dissect." Further, even very small causes (interference) can have large effects; that is, the cause-effect relationship is not linear. This was revealed by Edward Lorenz and Eustace Tilly who were attempting to do computer simulations of weather and found that even very small differences in initial conditions could result in very large changes in weather patterns. They called this the "Butterfly Effect," meaning that the beating of a butterfly's wings in one part of the world can change air flow patterns just enough so that tornadoes occur somewhere else.

23. Lack of funds has been and continues to be a problem. Apparently misinterpreting the methods and aims of our research, several of the major weight-loss organizations have declined to provide funding.

24. This is really a tentative statement, since at times we used professionals in our study and they seemed to be affected not at all by the presence of observers. No objection can be made to our using pros. Kinsey paid people for their sexual histories—"the economically poorer elements in the population, to persons who are professionally involved in sexual activities (as prostitutes, pimps, exhibitionists, etc.) or …others who have turned from their regular occupation and spend considerable time in helping make contacts"—and concludes that there "is no evidence that such payments have distorted the quality of the record…" (*Sexual Behavior in the Human Male, 27*).

25. Using professionals reduced our funds further.

26. There has been some questioning of our results based on our test group (too small) and our control group (none). Recently a scientific report received national attention: the "study" of two people revealed that we have a fat gene! Two people! A fat gene! As if obesity wasn't the result of complex interactions of genetics and conscious and unconscious actions, often determined (or at least circumscribed) by cultural factors. How can anyone claim that our sample was too small?

27. We have concealed the identities of the study participants by using pseudonyms throughout the book. We may be chastised by *Brill's Content* for using unnamed sources, but they must remain anonymous (none works for *Brill's* by the way).

28. These two subjects were enthusiastic and responsive—very valuable. We are pleased to report that they will be available again in ten to twenty-two months.

29. Although it is not considered desirable for the observers to assume the role of observed, we were scrupulous about factoring out personal biases. In any case our pre-study experiences in part provided the impetus for the study and our pre-study data contributed substantially to our conclusions (this book). We do not believe that our roles as observer-participants resulted in a conflicted experience.

30. There was one puzzling piece of data that we are unable to explain. It is conceivable that it is the result of a flaw in our method of measurement, but we just don't know at this point. In 89% of all sessions, the male subject immediately lost from 0.3 to 1.9 ounces more weight than the female subject. However, by the time of the next session, each male had regained from 79% to 107% of this lost weight.

31. We would have liked to have had stress tests administered more frequently, but the costs of the tests prohibited this.

32. Except the two professionals; see four notes back.

33. It is possible that her very positive response was due to the fees she received (she was one of the professionals) and her desire to "tell us what we wanted to hear." We do not believe this, but even if it were so, it would not negate the facts that she did lose weight and she certainly looked great.

34. This is a method frequently employed by *Consumer Reports*. In addition to putting products through numerous tests, they ask users (experts and ordinary consumers) their views about a product. Thus, for example, they can correlate the response of tasters of cheese with their laboratory analysis of cheese.

35. Due, of course, to lack of funding, not to any deliberate choice on our part or ignorance of scientific methods.

Appendix B

1. A complete investigation of the unknown side of Dickinson can be found in my book, *Emily Dickinson: Understood At Last!*, which will be published by Thalia Imprints in the near future. (Dr. Bathous is the recent winner of the Isaac Asimov Award for Quantitative Excellence and his *Musings of a Lifetime* is available in twelve-pound and twenty-two-pound editions. [ed.])

2. Poem 351. All quotations of her poetry are from *The Complete Poems of Emily Dickinson*, Thomas H. Johnson, ed. (Boston and Toronto: Little, Brown and Co., 1960), a reading version of the Harvard variorum text *The Poems of Emily Dickinson*,

3 vols. (Belknap Press, 1955). Dickinson did not title her poems; we use the numbers assigned by Johnson.

3. Walt Whitman, another erotic poet, says of the night, "Press close bare-bosom'd night—press close magnetic nourishing night!/ Night of south winds—night of the large few stars!/ Still nodding night—mad naked summer night" ("Song of Myself" #21).

4. She writes about her fears concerning the loss of her virginity in Poem 461:

> A Wife—at Daybreak I shall be—
> At Midnight, I am but a Maid,
> How short it takes to make a Bride—
> So soon to be a Child no more

5. Martha Dickinson Bianchi, *The Life and Letters of Emily Dickinson* (Boston and New York: Houghton Mifflin Co., 1924), 94. There is a new book *New Poems of Emily Dickinson* edited by Wm. H. Shurr (with Anna Dunlap and Emily Grey Shurr); they contend that Dickinson regularly embedded poems (over 500) disguised as prose in her letters. Maybe.

6. In Poem 383, Emily wrote this about Hunt:

> Exhilaration…
> To stimulate a Man
> Who hath the Ample Rhine
> Within his Closet—Best you can
> Exhale in offering

"Rhine" refers to the rhinoceros whose horn is a phallic symbol and used as an aphrodisiac. "Closet" is a slang term for men's trousers. And "Exhale" is a euphemism for fellatio.

7. Poem 612:

> It would have starved a Gnat—
> To live so small as I—
> And yet I was a living Child—
> With Food's necessity
> Upon me—Like a Claw—

She is referring here to psychological and emotional, not physiological, starvation.

8. She had at least one important homosexual experience, probably, as with most people, during her adolescence (Poem 631):

> Ourselves were wed one summer—dear—
> Your Vision—was in June—
> And overtaken in the Dark—
> Where You had put me down—
> 'Tis true—Our Futures different lay—
> 'Tis true, Your Garden led the Bloom,
> For mine—in Frosts—was sown—
> And yet, one Summer, we were Queens—
> But You—were crowned in June—

The experience was not very good for Emily, although her "friend" went on to prosper.

9. Bianchi says that "She was always in love with her teachers at that time, quite regardless of their being men or women..." (19). As late as when she was 50, in a poem given to her brother's children she wrote, "When He [Jesus] and I were Boys ..." (Poem 1487).

10. In a letter to Annie P. Strong (7 May 1845) she wrote: "I am growing handsome very fast indeed! I expect I shall be the belle of Amherst when I reach my 17th year. I don't doubt that I shall have perfect crowds of admirers at that age. Then how I shall delight to make them await my bidding, and with what delight shall I witness their suspense while I make my final decision" (Bianchi, 112).

11. One might argue that she could have broken the various "isms" that held her in bondage; that is, that given her wit, her intelligence and her writing ability she could have fled the restrictive environment of Amherst and made a place for herself in Boston or New York. Maybe. But to believe that you would have to believe that Hedda Gabler could have left George Tessman and gotten a job as a restaurant hostess.

12. For a time she undertook a study of world religions, but except for the Jehovah's Witnesses (Poem 626: "The Jehovahs—are no Babblers"), she found nothing good in any religion.

13. Incidentally, Bartlett's *Familiar Quotations* (14th edition) is wrong when it attributes the following lines to one of Dickinson's poems (when she was depressed about being overweight):

> Am I?—Can I be
> But a Dingleberry—
> Dangling—

In the Ass of God?

It looks like a Dickinson poem (she was so modern), but it was Richard Nixon who asked this of Henry Kissinger who replied, "I believe the correct preposition would be 'from' not 'in' Mr. President."

14. This did not bother her; in Poem 709 she writes:

> Publication—is the Auction
> Of the Mind of man—
> Poverty—be justifying
> For so foul a thing

We do not agree with her on this. P. B.

15. In Poem 709 she writes:

> …We—would rather
> From Our Garret go
> White—Unto the White Creator—
> Than invest—Our Snow

By "invest" she means make public (publish) her poems which reveal her inner true self.

16. In Poem 538 she says, "'Tis true—They shut me in the Cold—/ But then—Themselves were warm/ And could not know the feeling 'twas." And in Poem 540 she writes, "I took my Power in my Hand—/ And went against the World."

17. Poem 508:

> [T]oo small the first—
> A half unconscious Queen—
> But this time—Adequate—Erect

18. In her poetry she could even express her "radical" views toward mercy killing (Poem 908):

> 'Tis Sunrise—Little Maid…
> 'Tis Noon—My little Maid—
> My little Maid—'Tis Night…
> Had'st thou broached
> Thy little Plan to Die—
> Dissuade thee, if I could not, Sweet,

I might have aided—thee—

and necrophilia (Poem 611):

> I see thee better—in the Dark—
> I do not need a Light—
> The love of Thee—a Prism be—
> Excelling Violet—
> And in the Grave—I see Thee best—
> Its little Panels be
> Aglow—All ruddy—with the Light
> I held so high, for Thee

19. She writes in Poem 784:

> And when I sought my Bed—
> The Grave it was reposed upon
> The Pillow for my Head—
> I waked to find it first awake—
> I rose—It followed me—
> I tried to drop it in the Crowd—
> To lose it in the Sea—
> In Cups of artificial Drowse
> To steep its shape away—

20. Dickinson never married and her poetry tells us why. In Poem 944 she points out the difference between the male and female roles, especially in a marriage:

> I learned—at least—what Home could be—
> How ignorant I had been
> The Task for Both—
> When Play be done—
> Your problem—of the Brain—
> And mine—some foolisher effect—
> A Ruffle—or a Tune—

About the marriage vows she wrote: "Till Death—is narrow Loving" (Poem 907).
21. Poem 506: "And now, I'm different from before,/ As if I breathed superior air."

22. In her poetry, Dickinson could be not only frank but also raunchy as in this poem written about her friend Fanny Richardson on the occasion of a trip to the beach (Poem 507): "Ah, Pussy, of the Sand,/ The Hopes so juicy ripening—".

23. A number of composers have set Dickinson's songs to music: Aaron Copland, Alice Parker, Vincent Persichetti, Walter Hilse, Gitta Steiner, David Irving, Martin Kalmanoff, Quartilla Bovineio, Richard Hoyt. It is an interesting fact that almost all of her poems can be sung to the tune of "The Yellow Rose of Texas" and "The Battle Hymn of the Republic." Really! Try it.

Notes to the Notes

Chapter 2

a. They condemn what they do not understand. [ed.]

Chapter 6

a. Unfortunately, yesterday. We do not mean to imply that relations between men and women are universally enlightened today. But, in this country at least, there have been some significant positive changes.

b. Don't you just love passive constructions? By whom? C. F.

c. For example, men can now wear red pants, white shoes and their hair down over their ears or an earring without embarrassment. Achievements? Frittered? C. F.

d. *Screening History* (Cambridge, Mass.: Harvard Univ. Press, 1992), 59.

e. We have been receiving a lot of negative feedback from those we have approached about funding for our future studies; I am weary of the ignorant failing to see the usefulness of Swell-Wimp.

f. Listen to Christine Lavin's song "New-Age Guys."

Chapter 8

a. We say "physicians" (not "doctors") because they have medical degrees (MD) not Ph. D. (like ourselves). The term "doctor" or "medico" should be applied to those holding a doctorate and the term "physician" applied to those holding an MD which is NOT an academic degree, but a vocational degree (like a welder's certificate) the possessors of which require oversight by the state (a license) to maintain acceptable standards (as with hairdressers) and prevent fraud. In order to use a title you must earn it, pay your dues. I cannot call myself general, heavy-weight boxing champion, Pulitzer Prize winner (yet), mother or CPA because I haven't earned those titles. To become a general, physician, etc. you must follow the proscribed courses of education, testing and accumulate corollary experiences. MDs pay physician dues, not doctor dues. (Of course, it is possible to get an academic doctorate in several medical areas.) If you want to be called "doctor," get a doctorate (a real doctorate not something like a JD that pseudo-degree that lawyers claim entitles them to the title). Further, there are no equivalencies; you must earn the degree; those who call themselves "doctor" because they have been given an honorary doctorate are beneath contempt. I feel better now.

b. The original remark was made by boxer Robert Fitzsimmons before his match with James J. Jeffries (a heavier man) on 9 June 1899: "The bigger they come, the harder they fall."

Chapter 9

a. As Dave Barry says, you can't make this stuff up. I just received the October 1999 issue of *Consumer Reports* which contains an article on drugs and drugstores, "Relief for the Rx Blues" (38–44). In a survey of drugstores 16 of 25 pharmacists failed to warn of an adverse drug interaction (Coumadin and ginko biloba) even when asked a specific question (40). In order to increase profits some stores are thinking about "dispensing more medicine in prepackaged amounts instead of moving pills from big bottles to little ones" (40). (*Consumer Reports* doesn't point out that this will not result in lower prices for consumers; pre-packaged birth control pills are increasing in price.) In "1998 the industry attained a return on equity of nearly 40 percent" (41); no comment necessary. Finally, I was wrong in thinking that research and legal costs are the major contributors to drug prices: "the industry as a whole spends at least as much advertising and promoting drugs as it does developing them—and some major firms spend much more" (41).

Chapter 10

a. On September 7, 1921 Fatty Arbuckle accidentally ruptured Virginia Rappe's bladder while engaging in coitus in the missionary position.

b. Trans. H. T. Lowe-Porter (NY: The Modern Library, 1952), 264.

Chapter 14

a. This is a form of "birth control" that just happens to give pleasure to men but, at best, gives women no pleasure and usually pain. C. F.

b. We accept Reagan's aides' assurances that he was not suffering from Alzheimer's disease while in office.

c. It was quite a shock to celebrate my 50th birthday (and a celebration it was) and two days later receive a solicitation from AARP (and every six weeks or so since then). If their researchers can find out that I've passed 50, they should be able to determine whether I'm receiving Social Security benefits. I can't retire for another 12 years and if the politicians have their way I may not be able to retire for another 20 years. "Retired People" indeed! P. B.

d. If Sigmund Freud had never existed, the world today would be little different except for the absence of a lot of suffering and many bad books. His metaphor (which is all Freudian psychology is) provides no better understanding of the human mind than does astrology, the mind-as-complex-computer analogy or the various religious ideas of the mind/soul. That is, the paraphernalia of psychoanalysis (ego, id, oedipal complex, infantile sexuality, sublimation, transference, etceteras) is no more useful in treating a psychological problem than assuming a mind-transistor has burned out or the individual has been possessed by a malicious spirit. If he were alive and writing today, Freud would become the leader of a New Age sect and/or the darling of talk shows and TV "news magazines"; he would be shunned by academics and professionals. Paraphrasing Jacques Derrida, Freudian psychology always already was empty; oh, that we could put it *sous rature* (under erasure).[e] Of course, I'm no psychologist, but neither was Freud! As Lord Byron said to Lady Blessington when she complained about his denunciation of Thomas Moore, "Madam, I cannot stop. The fit is upon me."

e. See also "The Case of Silas Tomkyn Comerbach," by Captain Robert Tuttle in *Military Psychology*, ed. D. A. Sein (Paris: Blague, 1977).

Bibliography

Adams, Douglas. *The Hitchhiker's Guide to the Galaxy.* NY: Pocket Books, 1979.

Adler, T. "Impotence: More Than a Middle-age Metaphor." *Science News* 8 Jan. 1994, 21.

Andrews, Joseph and Pamela. *Chastity: Two Views.* Berlin: Prignitz and Scroderus, 1969.

Andreyich, Yakov. *The New Age Approach to Regularity.* NY: Pugidion Books, 1989.

Anthony, Catherine Parker. *Textbook of Anatomy and Physiology.* 6th ed. Saint Louis: C. V. Mosby, 1963.

Ard, Elizabeth. *Arms Control Development.* NY: Saurian Books, 1973.

Augustine, St. *The Confessions.* Trans. John K. Ryan. Garden City: Image Books, 1960.

Baker, Nicholson. *Vox.* NY: Random House, 1992.

Barrows, Plover. "The Psychology of Dieting." *NosuThryl: The Journal of Inner Plasma Studies* 12: 3–21.

Barth, John. *Lost in the Funhouse.* NY: Bantam Books, 1963.

Barth, John. *Tidewater Tales.* NY: G. P. Putnam's Sons, 1987.

Bell, T. *Kalogynomia: or the Laws of Female Beauty.* London: J. J. Stockdale, 1821.

Benengeli, Cide H. "The Impossible Dream." *Bedle's Monthly* March 1977, 54–59.

Barnard, Marie. *Sexual Deviations as Seen in Handwriting.* Genf: Ariston, 1994.

Bianchi, Martha Dickinson. *The Life and Letters of Emily Dickinson.* Boston & New York: Houghton Mifflin, 1924.

Birkel, Dee Ann Green, and Susan Birkel Freitag. *Forever Fit: A Step-By-Step Guide for Older Adults.* NY: Plenum Publishing, 1991.

Boccaccio, Giovanni. *The Decameron.* Trans. Richard Aldington. New York: Dell Publishing, 1930.

Boece, Hector and George Buchanan. *The Big Book of Sexual Positions.* Newgate: Rank Publishers, 1982.

Bonner, Elena. *Alone Together.* NY: A. A. Knopf, 1986.

Boorsicot, Bernard. *Shi Pei Pu: Pleasure Without Fear.* NY: Melpomene Books, 1992.

Bordo, Susan. *The Male Body.* NY: Farrar, Straus & Giraux, 1999.

"The Brain of a Glutton." *Discover* June 1992, 14–15.

Brennan, Karen. *Wild Desire.* Univ. of Massachusetts Press, 1991.

Brown, Walter A. "The Placebo Effect." *Scientific American* Jan. 1998, 90–95.

Bryson, Bill. *The Mother Tongue.* NY: William Morrow, 1990.

Busch, Heather and Burton Silver. *Kokigamii: The Intimate Art of the Little Paper Costume.* Berkeley: Ten Speed Press, 1992.

Busi, Aldo. *The Standard Life of a Temporary Pantyhose Salesman.* Italy, 1985; Britain, 1989.

Byrd, Richard E. *Alone.* NY: G. P. Putnam's Sons, 1938.

Caldwell, Mark. *A Short History of Rudeness.* NY: Picador, 1999.

Cambridge Companion to Buggery, The. NY: Cambridge Univ. Press, 1979.

Champollion, Jean-François. *It's as Easy as ABC.* Paris: Kunastrokius Press, 1992.

"Can You Live Longer?" *Consumer Reports* January 1992, 7–15.

"Can We live to 150?" *Popular Science* Nov. 1993, 77–82.

Caprio, Frank S. *The Sexually Adequate Female.* New York: Citadel Press, 1953.

"The cashews-and-cabbages diet melts pounds away!" *Ladies' Companion* 8 August 1984, 21.

Charnas, Suzy McKee. *Motherlines.* NY: Berkley Publishing, 1978.

Chaucer, Geoffrey. *The Tales of Canterbury.* Ed. Robert A. Pratt. Boston: Houghton Mifflin, 1974.

Chikatilo, Andrei. *Overcoming Food Aversions.* Moscow: Lutumilious Books, 1991. Cibber, Lewis and Colley Theobald. *The Lickerish Licorice.* Calliope, NJ: Paronomasia Ltd., 1969.

Clark, William R. *Time of Our Lives: the Science of Human Aging.* NY: Oxford Univ. Press, 1999.

Cleland, John. *Memoirs of a Woman of Pleasure.* New York: G. P. Putnam's Sons, 1963.

"Coitus." *Grove's Dictionary of Music and Musicians.* NY: St. Martin's Press, 1955.

Comfort, Alex. *The New Joy of Sex: A Gourmet Guide to Lovemaking for the Nineties.* New York: Crown Publishers, 1991.

Consumer Reports May 1993, 300.

Control Data Corporation. Internal Memorandum: H.K. to J.D. 23 May 1986.

"Couple Run Over By Train." *The Scranton Tribune* 31 June 1987, 5.

Crement, Xavier. *A**hole No More!: A Self-Help Guide for Recovering A**holes.* Canal Winchester, OH: Enthea Press, 1991.

Crews, Frederick. *The Poo Perplex.* NY: NAL-Dutton, 1965.

Cullen, William. *Nosology.* NY: Alan Sokal Imprints, 1991.

Danbrot, Margaret. *The New Cabbage Soup Diet.* NY: St. Martin's, 1997.

D'Eon, Chavalier. *Menage a trois—Why not?* Boston: Coituphilous Publications, 1972.

De Newman, Alfredo E. *Quid? Perturbabo?* Boggley Wollah: Pseudolus Imprints, 1987.

Denny, William. *Recreational Aspects of Sex and Mental Prophylaxis: A True Guide to Happiness.* Bremerhaven: Porter Books, 1931.

Dickens, Charles. *Bleak House.* Penguin Books, 1971.

Dickinson, Emily. *The Complete Poems of Emily Dickinson.* Ed. Thomas H. Johnson. Boston and Toronto: Little, Brown and Co., 1960.

Duncan, Barry L. and Joseph W. Rock. *Overcoming Relationship Impasses: Ways to Initiate Change When Your Partner Won't Help.* NY: Plenum Publishing, 1991.

Ehrlich, Eugene. *Amo, Amas, Amat and More.* New York: Harper & Row, 1985.

Eichel, Edward, and Philip Nobile. *The Perfect Fit: How to Achieve Mutual Fulfillment and Monogamous Passion Through the New Intercourse.* NY: Donald Fine, 1992.

Eichenbaum, Ken. *The Toilets of New York.* Milwaukee: Litterati Books, 1991.

Ekaf, Eman. "Fattening Foods To Avoid During The Holidays." *Redbook* December 1981, 67.

Empson, William. *Seven Types of Ambiguity.* NY: Noonday Press, 1955.

Erato, Euterpe. "Sooterkin Songs." *Chambre Syndicale de les Grandes Horizontales Americaine.* 69: 23–40.

Extra! March/April 1999, 22–24.

Fart Proudly: Writings of Benjamin Franklin You Never Read in School. Ed. Carl Japikse. Canal Winchester, OH: Enthea Press, 1991.

Fausto-Sterling, Anne. "Why Do We Know So Little About Human Sex?" *Discover* June 1992, 29–31.

Fitzgerald, Francis S. *This Side of Paradise.* NY: A. L. Burt, 1920.

Foucault, Michel. *The Order of Things.* NY: Vintage Books, 1973.

Forum Adviser: The Answers To Every Question You Ever Had About Sex. Penthouse Forum Magazine, 1977.

Freedman, David H. "The Aggressive Egg." *Discover* June 1992, 61–65.

Friedan, Betty. *The Feminine Mystique.* NY: Norton, 1963.

Gilman, Charlotte Perkins. *Herland.* NY: Pantheon Books, 1979.

Gladwell, Malcolm. "The Pima Paradox." *The New Yorker* 2 Feb. 1998, 44–57.

Glass, Stephen. "Sex Makes Me Sweat." *Hetaera* April 1983, 51–52.

Gochros, Harvey L. and Jean S. *The Sexually Oppressed.* New York: Associated Press, 1977.

Goldberg, Jonathan. *Sodometries.* Stanford Univ. Press, 1992.

Golden Book of Making Babies, The. Paris: Oulipo, 1945.

Golod, Kholod. *Living with the Glacier.* National Geographical Society, 1990.

Gotama, Siddhattha. *The Eightfold Road to Enlightenment.* Calcutta: Kalutas and Ganikas, 1982.

Greer, Germaine. *The Female Eunuch.* London: MacGibbon & Kee, 1970.

Groopman, Jerome. "Contagion." *The New Yorker* 13 September 1999, 34–49.

Hall, N. John. *Trollope.* NY: Oxford Univ. Press, 1991.

Hardy, Thomas. *The Mayor of Casterbridge.* Boston: Houghton Mifflin, 1962.

Harris, W. V. "Old Wives' Tales." *The New York Review of Books* 18 Nov. 1993, 52–54.

Heslinga, K. *Not Made of Stone: The Sexual Problems of Handicapped People.* Springfield, IL: Charles C. Thomas, 1974.

Himnia, Polly. "Build Your Own Ergometer." *Popular Mechanics* June 1983, 67–73.

Hitchens, Christopher. *The Missionary Position.* London & NY: Verso, 1996.

Hite, Shere. *The Hite Report: A Nationwide Study of Female Sexuality.* New York: Macmillan; London: Collier Macmillan, 1976.

Holman, C. Hugh. *A Handbook to Literature.* 3rd ed. Indianapolis: Bobbs-Merrill, 1972.

Honigmann, E. A. J. "The Second-Best Bed." *The New York Review of Books* November 7, 1991, 27–30.

Humbert, Humbert. *Confession of a White Widowed Male.* Paris: Olympia Press, 1955.

Humphry, Derek. *Final Exit.* Eugene, OR: The Hemlock Society, 1991.

Izdat, Sam. "The Sad End of Frau Drei Hummerbuns' Marriage." *Coprolites* November 1923, 65–69.

Jakes, Merda. *1001 Ways to Do It.* Drury Lane Imprints, 1978.

Jones, James H. *Alfred C. Kinsey: A Public/Private Life.* NY: W. W. Norton, 1997.

Kael, Pauline. *Kiss Kiss, Bang Bang.* Boston: Little Brown, 1968.

Kama Sutra of Vatsyayan, The. Trans. Richard Burton & F. F. Arbuthnot. New York: Capricorn Books, 1963.

King, Stephen. *Gerald's Game.* NY: Viking, 1992.

Kinnell, Galway. *When One has Lived a Long Time Alone.* NY: Knopf, 1991.

Kinsey, Alfred C., Wardell B. Pomeroy and Clyde E. Martin. *Sexual Behavior in the Human Male.* Philadelphia & London: W. B. Saunders, 1948.

Kinsey, Alfred C., Wardell B. Pomeroy, Clyde E. Martin, and Paul H. Gebhard. *Sexual Behavior in the Human Female.* Philadelphia & London: W. B. Saunders, 1953.

Kirkwood, Tom. *A Means to an End: The Biological Basis of Aging and Death.* NY: Oxford Univ. Press, 1999.

Lamber, Daniel. "Ergs and Nooky." *The Athletic Director.* The Hague: Poep & Stront, 1967.

Lancaster, Don. "The ISMM Revisited (II)." *Midnight Engineering* Sept/Oct 1991, 62.

Lane, Harley Warwick. "Sexual Activity and the Middle-Aged By-Pass Patient." *The Journal of Near, Far and North-by-North Eastern Yonic Studies* 10:78–94.

Lane, Margaret. *Purely for Pleasure* London: H. Hamilton, 1966.

Lee, Shelton Jackson. "Mo' Better Sex." *People* 13 June 1985, 23.

Leonoweng, Anna. *The Romance of the Harem.* Ed. Susan Morgan. Charlottesville: Univ. Press of Vrigina, 1991.

Leutwyler, Kristin. "Don't Stress." *Scientific American* Jan. 1998, 30.

Lisp, Franz. "Hungarian Notation." *Programmer's Update* July 1990, 18–35.

"Lose 5 pounds a week eating only facial tissues!" *The Tatler* 16 March 1989.

"Losing Weight: What Works. What Doesn't." *Consumer Reports* June 1993, 347–352.

"Low-Back Pain." *Scientific American* August 1998, 52.

Maines, Rachel P. *The Technology of Orgasm.* The John Hopkins Univ. Press, 1999.

Mann, Thomas. *The Magic Mountain.* Trans. H. T. Lowe-Porter. NY: The Modern Library, 1952.

Mardian, Alexas. *The Most Unkindest Cuts of All.* NY: Mohel Books, 1989.

Marquez, Garcia Gabriel. *100 Years of Solitude.* Trans. Gregory Rabassa. NY: Avon Books, 1970.

Masters, William H., and Virginia E. Johnson. *Human Sexual Inadequacy.* Boston: Little, Brown and Co., 1970.

Masters, William H., Virginia E. Johnson and Robert C. Kolodny. *On Sex and Human Loving.* Boston & Toronto: Little, Brown and Co., 1982.

Masters, William H., and Virginia E. Johnson. *Sexual Response.* Boston: Little Brown and Co., 1966.

McCarthy, Colman. "The Politics of Bicycling," *Liberal Opinion Week* 28 December 1992.

McMack, Ian. *Gaelic Etymologies.* New York: J. S. G. Boggs, 1990.

Midgley Jr., Thomas. *They Seemed Like Good Ideas at the Time.* Detroit: GM Books, 1997.

Nabokov, Vladimir. *Ada or Ardor: A Family Chronicle.* NY: McGraw-Hill, 1960.

Nabokov, Vladimir. *Glory.* Trans. Dimitri Nabokov. NY: McGraw-Hill, 1971.

Nabokov, Vladimir. *King. Queen, Knave.* NY: McGraw-Hill, 1968.

Nabokov, Vladimir. *Transparent Things.* NY: McGraw-Hill, 1972.

National Institute of Hemiplegia. *Publication* 217. n. p., 1979, 23.

Nayika, Lynn Gahm. "Sweating." *Encyclopaedia Sexualis.* Piltdown: Scitan Books, 1979.

Nemouicheck, Leonid. *In Search of the Perfect Orgasm.* Hafen: Momzer & Towzer, 1989.

"New electronic device flattens tummies in 2 minutes!" *Household Words* 1 January 1981.

Nietzsche, Friedrich. *Thus Spoke Zarathustra.* Trans. Walter Kaufmann. Harmondsworth: Penguin Books, 1978.

Nordic Row TBX Advertisement. *The New Yorker* 16 April 1991, 32.

Nordic Trac Advertisement. *The New Yorker* 2 Sept. 1991, 69.

O'Donnell, Mark. *Vertigo Park.* NY: Alfred A. Knopf, 1993.

One Hundred Years After Tomorrow. Ed. and trans. Darlene J. Sadlier. Indiana Univ. Press, 1991.

"The Pain Perplex." *The New Yorker* 21 Sept. 1998, 88.

Phillips, Adam. *Kissing, Tickling and Being Bored.* Cambridge, Mass.: Harvard Univ. Press, 1993.

Pietropinto, Anthony, and Jacqueline Simenauer. *Beyond the Male Myth: What Women Want to Know about Men's Sexuality.* New York: Times Books, 1977.

Plunkett, James. *Strumpet City.* NY: Dell, 1969.

Pope, Alexander. *Poetry and Prose of Alexander Pope.* Ed. Aubrey Williams. Boston: Houghton Mifflin, 1969.

Pope, Popadià, and Athole Athwiper. *National Health Care and the Self-Employed.* Thule: Boinkmeister, 1986.

Proust, Madeleine. "Diet and the Elderly Neurasthenic." *The Chirurgical Journal* 56: 237–252

Quarterly Review of Doublespeak April 1993, 5.

Rabener, Gottlieb Wilhelm. *Hinknars von Repkow: Noten ohne Text.* Berlin: U. N. Heimlich, 1743.

Ray, Jr., John. "She Couldn't Stay Small." *Cornell Studies* 54:112–119.

"Relief for the Rx Blues." *Consumer Reports* October 1999, 38–44.

Reuben, David. *Everything You Always Wanted to Know About Sex But Were Afraid to Ask.* New York: Bantam Books, 1969.

Resurgam, Peter. *Damaged Goods.* Paris: Eugène Brieux, 1903.

Roach, Mary. "Intimate Engineering." *Discover* Feb.1999.

Rudolf, Val and Tina. *The Shrieking Chic Sheik.* Sterocorceous, NY: Sirreverence Books, 1923.

Rumfoord, Bertram Copeland. *Sex and Athletics for the Senior Male.* Ilium, NY: Dresden Books, 1945.

Rush, Norman. *Mating.* NY: A.A. Knopf, 1991.

Sapolsky, Robert. "Growing Up in a Hurry." *Discover* June 1992.

Schiller, Lawrence. "Justice Boulder Style." *The New Yorker* 19 Jan. 1998, 32–37.

Schor, Juliet B. *The Overworked American: The Unexpected Decline of Leisure.* NY: Basic Books, 1992.

Sélavy, Rrose, and Sheila Taque. *The Economic Factor and the Health of Sex Professionals.* Detroit: Ouslan Press, 1977.

Shakespeare, William. *The Riverside Shakespeare.* Boston: Houghton Mifflin Co., 1974.

Showalter, Elaine. *Sexual Anarchy: Gender and Culture at the Fin de Siècle.* NY: Penguin USA, 1991.

Small, Meredith F. "What's Love Got to Do With It?" *Discover* June 1992, 48–49.

Stephensen, Mary. *My Child Is a Mother.* San Antonia: Corona Publishing, 1992.

Sterne, Laurence. *Tristram Shandy.* Indianapolis: The Odysses Press, 1940.

"Straight Sex and AIDS Vaccines." *Discover* January 1992.

Swift, Dean. *A Tale of a Tub.* London: John Nutt, 1973.

Swinburne, A. C. *Lesbia Brandon.* London: Falcon Press, 1952.

Thackery, William. *Vanity Fair.* 1848; Harmondsworth: Penguin Books, 1968.

Titorenko, Raisa Maksimovna. *I Hope.* Trans. David Floyd. NY: Harper Collins, 1991.

Tomizza, Fulvio. *Heavenly Supper: The Story of Maria Janis.* Univ. of Chicago Press, 1991.

"Top-selling diets." *Consumer Reports* Jan. 1998, 60.

Trilling, Lionel. *Liberal Imagination.* Garden City, NY: Doubleday, 1953.

Tuttle, Robert. "The Case of Silas Tomkyn Comerbach." *Military Psychology.* Ed. D. A. Sein. Paris: Blague, 1977.

Tylutki, George. "An Invalid But Useful Analogy." *Computer Language* July 1991, 119–120.

Tylutki, George. "What Good is *self?*" *Computer Language* May 1989, 34–47.

United States Department of Health, Education and Welfare. *The Homemaker's Calorie Chart.* GPO: 1982.

Veen, Adelaida and Ivan. *Ardor in Ardis.* n.p.: Cunnus-Coglione Books, 1923.

Vestey, Michael. "Decent Into Tackiness." *The Spectator* 27 March 1999, 51–52.

Vidal, Gore. *Myron.* NY: Random House, 1974.

Vidal, Gore. *Screening History.* Cambridge, Mass.: Harvard Univ. Press, 1992.

Von Kreisler, Kristin. "The Healing Powers of Sex." *Reader's Digest* June 1993.

Waite, Q. and I. Racque. *A Case Study: Warba & Bubiyan After the Attacks.* Berlin: Waswill Dasweib, 1992.

Wallechinsky, David, Irving Wallace, and Amy Wallace. *The Book of Lists.* New York: Bantam Books, 1977.

Wills, Garry. "Athena's Magic." *The New York Review of Books* 17 December 1992, 50.

Wirtz, Billy C. *The Missionary Position.* Raleigh, NC: n.p., 1993.

Wise, Thomas J. *The Illustrated Victorian Sex Manual.* Marshalsea: Stews and Bagnios, 1889.

Wright, Karen. "Evolution of the Big O." *Discover* June 1992, 53–58.

Yana, V. Atsya. "A Caber a Day Keeps the Doctor Away." *Sports Medicine* 12:321–44.

Yana, V. Atsya. *Geriatric Weightlifting.* New York: Bumfodden, 1979.

Zi'Peppe, Giuli. *Twelve Steps to Self Confidence.* Warsaw: Benkart, 1988.

Zola, Émile. *Nana.* Trans. George Holden. Baltimore: Penguin Books, 1972.

Zulo, Harold. "Pessimistic Rumination in Popular Songs and News Magazines Predict Economic Recession Via Decreased Consumer Optimism and Spending." *Journal of Economic Psychology* 1991.

Zwiep, Mary. *Pilgrim Path: The First Company of Women Missionaries to Hawaii.* Univ. of Wisconsin Press, 1992.

www.ingramcontent.com/pod-product-compliance
Lightning Source LLC
Chambersburg PA
CBHW030424290526
45786CB00001B/134